Human Metapneumovirus (HMPV) in 2025

Azhar ul Haque Sario

Copyright

First Printing, 2025

Azhar.sario@hotmail.co.uk

Disclaimer: This book is free from AI use. The cover was designed in Microsoft Publisher

Disclaimer: The author has no affiliation with any official board or entity related to Human Metapneumovirus diagnostics, treatment guidelines, or vaccine development. This work is independently produced under nominative fair use for informational purposes.

Contents

HMPV Unveiled: Discovery, Molecular Identity, and Enduring Relevance

The Ghost in the Machine: Unmasking HMPV, the Respiratory Phantom We Didn't Know We Were Fighting

Imagine the scene, repeated countless times in clinics and hospitals across decades: a child wheezing, struggling for breath, maybe an elderly patient battling a harsh cough that settles deep in their chest. Doctors run the tests for the usual suspects – Respiratory Syncytial Virus (RSV), influenza – but the results come back negative. Yet, the illness is undeniably real, sometimes severe. It was a medical mystery playing out in plain sight, a significant chunk of respiratory misery attributed to... well, something unknown. A viral ghost haunted the wards.

For years, this phantom eluded capture. Our standard method for nabbing viruses – coaxing them to grow in lab dishes (cell cultures) and watching for the tell-tale damage they inflict – was like trying to catch smoke with tweezers. This particular virus, we later learned, was a diva in the lab. Human Metapneumovirus (HMPV), as it would eventually be named, was incredibly fussy, growing slowly, poorly, or sometimes not at all in the usual cellular hotels, leaving behind only the faintest, most ambiguous clues. Trying to isolate it felt like chasing shadows.

Then, around the turn of the millennium, the game changed. A new generation of molecular tools emerged, acting like incredibly sensitive listening devices. Instead of needing a whole army of viruses grown in a dish, these techniques, particularly the powerhouse known as RT-PCR, could detect the faintest genetic whispers – tiny fragments of the virus's RNA – directly in a patient's sample. It was like finally having a flashlight powerful enough to pierce the gloom.

In 2001, researchers in the Netherlands pointed this flashlight into the darkness. Investigating those perplexing RSV-negative respiratory samples from sick children, they hit genetic gold. Using clever molecular strategies, they amplified and identified pieces of a virus unlike the usual suspects, belonging to the paramyxovirus family. The ghost finally had a name: Human Metapneumovirus. It wasn't just a discovery; it was a revelation, proving that our old ways of looking for viruses had left blind spots, and that the molecular age could illuminate pathogens previously cloaked in invisibility. The new PCR tests weren't just better; they were often the only way to reliably "see" HMPV, quickly becoming the detective's go-to tool.

But this discovery sparked an immediate, tantalizing question: Was HMPV a brand-new menace, freshly emerged to plague humanity? Or had it been walking among us all along, a silent, unrecognized member of our microbial landscape?

The answers came swiftly, like uncovering buried history. Scientists became molecular archaeologists. They pulled out old, frozen blood samples – time capsules of immunity dating back as far as 1958. Testing these decades-old serums, they found unmistakable footprints: antibodies specifically targeting HMPV. Our grandparents' and great-grandparents' immune systems had met, fought, and remembered this virus long before we even knew its name! Further digging unearthed HMPV's actual genetic material (RNA) hiding in archived respiratory specimens collected way back in the 1970s.

The verdict was clear: HMPV wasn't a newcomer. It was an old foe, a long-established human pathogen that had likely been causing coughs, colds, and serious respiratory infections for generations, maybe even centuries. It wasn't that the virus was new; our ability to finally see it was.

So where did this ancient companion come from? By comparing HMPV's genetic blueprint to known viruses, scientists found its closest relative: Avian Metapneumovirus (AMPV), a virus known to trouble birds, especially turkeys. This strongly suggested HMPV began as a bird virus that, at some point deep in the past – potentially hundreds of years ago – made the leap into humans. It wasn't a sudden, dramatic jump, but likely a slow burn, allowing the virus ample time to adapt to its new human hosts and spread across the globe, undetected.

From Ghost Story to Game Plan: What Knowing HMPV Changed

Unmasking HMPV wasn't just about solving a scientific puzzle; it had immediate, real-world consequences:

Clearing the Fog in Clinics: Doctors finally had a name for that frustrating "mystery virus." Reliable HMPV tests could be added to diagnostic panels. Imagine a pediatric ward during winter surge: knowing whether a child has RSV, the flu, or HMPV allows doctors to group patients properly (stopping spread), avoid pointless antibiotics (it's a virus!), and manage care much more precisely. Diagnosis went from a shrug to a specific answer.

Pinpointing Outbreak Culprits: Think of a respiratory outbreak ripping through a nursing home. If flu and RSV tests were negative, it used to be a dead end. Now, public health officials can specifically test for HMPV. Identifying it as the cause allows for targeted infection control – isolation, hygiene protocols – tailored to stop this specific virus, making outbreak management far more effective.

Mapping the True Enemy: Before 2001, HMPV's impact was invisible in public health data. Now, we can track it. We know it tends to peak in late winter and spring, often following the RSV wave. We know it's everywhere. Crucially, we know it's a major player, responsible for a significant slice (estimated 5-15%) of hospitalizations for lung infections in young kids, and a serious threat to the elderly and those with weakened immune systems. This knowledge helps allocate resources and anticipate seasonal surges.

Giving Hope a Target: You can't fight an enemy you can't see. Identifying HMPV gave scientists a clear target for developing weapons against it. While we don't have a licensed vaccine or specific antiviral drug yet, the discovery ignited the research engine. Scientists are actively studying HMPV's vulnerabilities, designing candidate vaccines, and testing potential treatments – work that simply couldn't have happened before 2001.

The unmasking of HMPV is a powerful reminder that the world of microbes is full of secrets, and that scientific progress, particularly the leap into molecular tools, can suddenly bring long-hidden truths into sharp focus. It turned a respiratory phantom into a known entity, transforming how we diagnose illness, manage outbreaks, understand disease patterns, and work towards a healthier future. The ghost is still out there, but now, we can see it coming.

HMPV: Finding its Tribe - How a Viral Misunderstanding Changed Everything

Picture the bustling, invisible world of viruses like a sprawling, ancient city with distinct neighborhoods. For a long time, we thought Human Metapneumovirus (HMPV) – a notorious character known for causing respiratory grief, especially for little kids and the elderly – lived downtown in the massive Paramyxoviridae district, neighbors with big names like Measles and Mumps. It seemed to fit, kinda. But science, like a relentless detective, keeps getting better tools. Armed with sharper eyes (electron microscopes) and the ability to read molecular blueprints (genomics), scientists started noticing things about HMPV that just didn't quite match the neighbors.

It was like looking at a family portrait and realizing one person, while clearly related, had distinctly different features. The whispers grew louder until 2016, when the viral city planners – the ICTV – made a bold rezoning decision. They carved out a whole new district, Pneumoviridae, and declared that was HMPV's true home (specifically, on Metapneumovirus street within that district). This wasn't just rearranging nameplates; it was acknowledging HMPV belonged to a different tribe altogether, with its own unique customs and biology.

The Telltale Clues: More Than Skin Deep

What tipped the scales? It turns out, tribes have tells:

The "Build" Difference (Morphology): Zoom in close, really close, with those powerful microscopes. You see the virus's core structure, its nucleocapsid – think of it like the protective casing for its genetic instructions. The old neighbors in Paramyxoviridae central had a chunkier build, about 18 nanometers wide. But HMPV and its closer cousin, Respiratory Syncytial Virus (RSV, who lives on Pneumovirus street in the same new district), sported a slimmer profile, only 13-14 nm wide. A subtle difference? To a virus, that's like the difference between wearing chainmail and a sleek stealth suit – a fundamental design choice pointing to a separate evolutionary path.

Reading the "Instruction Manual" (Genomics): This was the clincher. Viruses like HMPV carry their entire operational plan in an RNA molecule.

Blueprint Layout (Gene Order): Imagine the RNA as an instruction manual. While all these viruses use similar types of instructions (genes for proteins like N, P, M, F, L etc.), the order they're written in matters. The Paramyxoviridae folks had one standard layout. But HMPV and RSV shared a different, distinct layout specific to their Pneumoviridae tribe. HMPV's specific sequence (3'-N-P-M-F-M2-SH-G-L-5') is its unique tribal dialect, slightly different even from RSV's, marking them as distinct but related families within the same tribe.

Missing Tools (The NS1/NS2 Gap): Here's a fascinating twist. Many viruses carry extra tools – non-structural proteins like NS1 and NS2 – specifically designed to sabotage the host's security systems (the immune response). Think of them as lock picks or jamming devices. The Paramyxoviridae crew often has these. But HMPV? It travels light. It lacks these specific NS1/NS2 tools. This isn't just missing equipment; it fundamentally changes how HMPV interacts with our bodies compared to its old, presumed relatives. Interestingly, even its closer cousin RSV does have NS1/NS2, highlighting that even within the Pneumoviridae district, HMPV's Metapneumovirus family has its own unique evolutionary strategies.

Why This Viral Genealogy Matters Right Now (in 2025)

Okay, so scientists rearranged the viral family tree. Why should anyone outside a lab care? Because this "correct address" is crucial for how we fight back:

Knowing Your Enemy: Just knowing HMPV is an "enveloped RNA virus" in the Pneumoviridae family tells us its basic vulnerabilities. Its fatty outer layer (envelope) means disinfectants work well. Its reliance on its own copying machine (the L protein) makes that machine a prime target for drugs. It's like knowing your opponent wears flammable clothing and relies on a single, unique weapon.

Spotting the Intruder (Diagnostics): When winter hits and emergency rooms fill with coughing, wheezing patients, doctors face a viral soup – could it be HMPV, RSV, flu, or something else? Precise identification is key. Thanks to knowing HMPV's unique genetic fingerprint (including the absence of NS1/NS2!), modern diagnostic tests (those sophisticated multiplex PCR panels you hear about) can rapidly pick HMPV out of the lineup.

Picture This (2025): A pediatric ward sees a surge in babies with severe lung inflammation (bronchiolitis). A quick molecular test, designed using this exact taxonomic knowledge, identifies a cluster of HMPV cases separate from an RSV outbreak down the hall. This lets staff group patients smartly to prevent cross-infection and guides care, especially since RSV has specific antibody treatments (like palivizumab for prevention) that HMPV currently doesn't. Knowing HMPV is responsible for a significant chunk (5-15%) of these hospitalizations makes accurate ID non-negotiable.

Designing Smarter Weapons (Therapy & Vaccines): Understanding HMPV's specific parts list is guiding the hunt for effective treatments.

The "F" protein is the key HMPV uses to break into our cells. Scientists are working hard to design vaccines and antibody therapies that jam this key or target it for destruction, learning from similar strategies against its cousin, RSV.

That unique viral copying machine, the "L" protein? It's a top target for custom-designed antiviral drugs that could shut down HMPV production specifically.

And critically, knowing HMPV lacks NS1/NS2 means scientists won't waste time developing drugs against those phantom targets – a strategy that might work for RSV or other viruses, but would be useless here.

Picture This (2025): An elderly resident in a care home gets severe pneumonia. Rapid testing confirms HMPV. While specific HMPV antivirals are still limited, this clear diagnosis rules out bacterial infection (requiring antibiotics) or flu (requiring different antivirals). It ensures proper supportive care and infection control. Perhaps this patient even qualifies for a clinical trial testing a new drug specifically designed to block HMPV's F or L protein – a trial made possible only by understanding the virus's precise identity and toolkit.

The Takeaway:

Giving HMPV its proper taxonomic address in the Pneumoviridae family wasn't just scientific housekeeping. It was unlocking a deeper understanding based on its physical build, its unique genetic instruction manual, and the tools it does (and doesn't) carry. Standing here in 2025, this clarity is fundamental. It shapes how we recognize HMPV in sick patients, how we track its spread, and most importantly, how we intelligently design the therapies and vaccines needed to protect the vulnerable from this widespread respiratory foe. Knowing its true identity is the first, crucial step in winning the fight.

The Shape-Shifting Traveler

Imagine trying to describe a cloud – it's mostly round, but not quite, right? Enveloped viruses are a bit like that. We call it pleomorphism. They don't stick to one rigid shape, often appearing as tiny spheres, sometimes stretching into threads, sometimes delightfully irregular (Ref 1). Picture a bustling crowd where everyone's roughly the same size (a minuscule 150 to 600 nanometers across!), yet each has their own subtle variation (Ref 1). It took powerful tools like cryo-electron microscopes – think ultra-powerful freeze-frame cameras – to truly appreciate this fluid identity, revealing that even viruses from the same "family" don't always look identical.

Dressed in Borrowed Finery: The Envelope and its Tools

Wrapping this tiny vessel is a lipid envelope, a soft outer layer. But here's the crafty part: the virus doesn't make this coat itself. It steals it, snatching a piece of the host cell's own membrane on its way out the door, like a thief grabbing a cloak during an escape (Evidence: Lab analysis shows the virus's coat perfectly matches the host cell's membrane lipids).

Studded onto this borrowed cloak are the virus's crown jewels: the glycoprotein spikes (Ref 1). These aren't just decorations; they're the essential tools for breaking and entering. Think of them as molecular grappling hooks and master keys, typically 13-17 nm long (Ref 1).

Two key players here are the Attachment (G) and Fusion (F) proteins (Ref 5, 1). The G protein often acts like a scout, searching for and latching onto the right "docking port" (receptor) on a potential host cell (Evidence: Scientists have mapped exactly where G proteins grab onto cells, like finding the specific keyhole). Once docked, the F protein takes center stage. It undergoes a dramatic shape-change, like a coiled spring releasing. It first harpoons the host cell membrane and then forcefully pulls the virus and cell together, merging their membranes and allowing the virus's internal contents to spill into the cell (Evidence: Stunning molecular snapshots show the F protein before and after it springs into action, revealing how it cracks open the door, Ref 5). Because these G and F proteins are on the outside and absolutely vital for invasion, they're the prime targets our immune system learns to recognize, and the bullseye for most vaccine designs (Ref 5, 1).

Real-World Impact (RSV Vaccine): Remember the F protein, the membrane-merging tool? Scientists figured out its exact shape before it springs into action. This "pre-fusion" shape turned out to be the perfect thing to show our immune system. Vaccines built around this specific shape trigger incredibly powerful antibodies that stop the RSV virus cold, far better than older approaches. This discovery, born from intricate molecular detective work, led directly to highly effective RSV vaccines now protecting vulnerable populations. Structure really is destiny here!

The Precious Cargo Within: The Nucleocapsid

Beneath the stolen cloak lies the virion's core: the nucleocapsid. For many enveloped RNA viruses, this is a beautifully organised helix (Ref 10). The virus's genetic instructions, its RNA genome, aren't just rattling around loose. Instead, the fragile RNA strand is snugly wrapped by countless copies of the Nucleoprotein (N) (Ref 10, 7). Imagine a delicate thread meticulously wound with protective beads – that's the N protein shielding the RNA. This tightly wound N-RNA complex (the ribonucleoprotein or RNP) acts like a secure vault, protecting the precious genetic code while also keeping it ready for copying once inside a host cell (Evidence: Experiments confirm N protein's role as RNA's bodyguard and organiser, Ref 7). The N protein is often one of the most plentiful components in the whole virion.

Real-World Impact (Rapid Tests): Why are those rapid COVID or flu tests often so fast? They frequently target this N protein. Because there's so much of it and its structure is fairly consistent even between different strains, it makes a great, easy-to-detect marker. Antibodies in the test strip latch onto any N protein present in your sample, giving a quick yes/no answer. Knowing the virion's contents directly enables rapid diagnostics!

The Engine Room: The Polymerase Complex

Tucked in with the protected RNA is the virus's own replication machinery – the polymerase complex. This is the engine that will drive the production of more viruses. Its main components are the Large protein (L), which holds the crucial RNA-copying enzyme (the RNA-dependent RNA polymerase or RdRp), and the Phosphoprotein (P), acting as an essential co-pilot, helping the L protein work efficiently and interact with the N-RNA template (Evidence: Genetic tweaks and biochemical tests pinpointed L and P's jobs, and advanced imaging is now showing how they physically work together on the RNA template). This dynamic duo reads the viral RNA, churning out both full-length copies for new virions and shorter messenger RNAs (mRNAs) that instruct the hijacked host cell to build viral proteins.

Real-World Impact (Antiviral Drugs): Since the L protein's copying function is absolutely essential for the virus and distinct from our own cellular machinery, it's a prime target for antiviral drugs. Scientists use detailed structural maps of the L protein's active site – the business end of the enzyme – to design molecules that specifically gum up its works. Drugs aiming to block this viral copy machine (like Remdesivir, which hits the RdRp of several viruses) are a direct result of understanding this core piece of the virion's architecture and its critical function.

The Masterpiece of Efficiency

So, the virion isn't just a random collection of parts. It's an incredibly efficient package. The envelope and spikes handle finding and entering the target. The nucleocapsid protects the vital genetic code. The polymerase complex waits, ready to execute the replication plan. Decoding this intricate interplay between structure and function, this molecular choreography, is more than just fascinating science. It's our roadmap to identifying vulnerabilities, designing smarter diagnostic tools, and creating targeted weapons – vaccines and antivirals – to disrupt the mission of these microscopic architects and protect us from the diseases they cause.

Imagine this virus not just as a pathogen, but as a tiny, incredibly efficient survival machine. Its entire operating system isn't written in the sturdy, double-stranded DNA we rely on, but on a single, delicate ribbon of RNA. Think of it like a fragile cassette tape, about 13,300 characters long [Fact/Figure], holding the essential instructions for viral existence (Ref 10, 5). This isn't just a jumble of code; it's meticulously organized in a specific sequence - a molecular recipe listed as 3′ -N-P-M-F-M2(1/2)-SH-G-L-5′ (Ref 10, 5). That's the precise order the virus reads to build everything it needs.

From this compact script, the virus conjures up its entire toolkit: a cast of just nine key proteins [Fact/Figure] (Ref 10, 5). Meet the players: 'N' (Nucleocapsid) lovingly wraps the precious RNA core. 'P' (Phosphoprotein) and 'L' (Large polymerase) are the copy machines, replicating the RNA. 'M' (Matrix) acts like the structural scaffolding. 'F' (Fusion) is the master key, prying open host cells. 'G' (Attachment) is the grappling hook, latching onto targets. Then there are the specialists: 'M2-1' and 'M2-2' fine-tuning the copying process, and 'SH' (Small Hydrophobic), a bit player whose exact role is still being fully understood (Ref 10, 5). The coordinated performance of this nine-protein ensemble is the virus's entire strategy for invasion, replication, and escape.

But here's where it gets really interesting: this virus is a relentless innovator, a master of disguise. It's not one single entity but exists as a diverse family with significant variations across the globe. Scientists have found it fundamentally splits into two major "clans," dubbed Genotype A and Genotype B (Ref 2). What drives this family feud? It largely comes down to changes in the genes for those 'F' (Fusion) and 'G' (Attachment) proteins – the very parts the virus shows to the outside world, its "face" and "hands," if you will (Ref 2). Changing these is like changing its coat and handshake, making it recognizable or unfamiliar to our immune system.

Digging deeper, researchers act like molecular genealogists, tracing even finer "family lines" or lineages within the A and B clans – think A1, A2a/b, B1, B2 (Ref 2). They track these subtle variations, often concentrated in those revealing F and G genes, mapping the virus's evolutionary journey in near real-time (Ref 2). It's like watching micro-evolution unfold season by season.

And the virus doesn't just sit still; it actively tinkers with its own code. Scientists have caught it in the act of making mistakes that stick, like accidentally duplicating parts of its 'G' gene (the grappling hook) in certain strains (Ref 11).

Imagine hitting "copy-paste" on a key feature – this could potentially change how the virus attaches to cells or how well our immune system recognizes it (Ref 11). We've literally witnessed entirely new viral lineages emerge and sweep across continents, showcasing its powerful ability to adapt and thrive (Ref 13).

This genetic restlessness isn't just academic curiosity; it has huge real-world consequences:

Catching the Culprit (Diagnostics): Knowing whether you're dealing with Clan A or B, or a specific lineage, is vital for accurate detective work [Application/Case Study]. Diagnostic tests, like the sophisticated PCR molecular photocopiers, need to be smart. They must target parts of the viral recipe book that either never change, or they must be specifically designed to spot the known differences (like A vs. B). Otherwise, a sneaky new variant might slip past undetected (Ref 2). Think of public health labs constantly checking the virus's genetic "fingerprints" to see which versions are causing trouble this season [Real-time Case Study].

The Master of Disguise (Immune Evasion): Those constant tweaks, especially to the 'G' and 'F' proteins on its surface, are the virus's secret weapon for immune evasion – a phenomenon called antigenic drift (Ref 2, 6). It's like the virus subtly changing its outfit [Application/Case Study]. Even if you've fought it off before, your immune system's "memory" might not fully recognize the slightly altered new version. This is the frustrating reason why we can catch this virus multiple times – it keeps changing just enough to sneak past our defenses (Ref 6).

The Vaccine Challenge (Vaccine Development): This constant shape-shifting poses the biggest hurdle for vaccines (Ref 7). A vaccine designed perfectly against one version (say, an older Genotype A strain) might not work as well against a newer Genotype B strain or an evolved lineage [Application/Case Study]. It's like having a key for only one door when the virus keeps changing the locks. The holy grail for researchers now is to design smarter vaccines: perhaps ones that train our immune system to recognize the parts of the virus that don't change easily, or maybe "multi-key" vaccines that include bits from both the A and B clans, offering broader protection against this ever-evolving foe (Ref 7).

So, while its genetic script is short (~13.3 kb RNA) and its protein toolkit small (just nine players), this virus packs a punch through its incredible diversity and adaptability. Understanding its family tree (genotypes A/B, lineages), its evolutionary tricks (like gene duplication), and its knack for changing its appearance (antigenic drift) is absolutely essential. This knowledge isn't just data; it's our roadmap for building better diagnostics, anticipating its evasive maneuvers, and ultimately, designing vaccines that can truly keep pace with this restless microscopic survivor.

The Intracellular Lifecycle: HMPV Replication Strategies and Host Cell Interactions

The First Hello: More Like Bumping into a Sticky Wall

Think of our virus, perhaps one like those behind mumps or RSV, initially bumping around the cell's neighborhood. Its first move isn't always a sophisticated lock-pick. Often, it uses what's called the 'G protein'. Picture this G protein as being covered in shaggy, sugary camouflage – it looks a bit different every time. Its go-to strategy? Just latching onto the cellular equivalent of fuzzy velcro strips plastered all over the building's exterior – these are GAGs (glycosaminoglycans). It's less of a targeted entry and more like sticking to the first available surface, hoping to get close enough to the real door. It's a way to hang around, increasing the odds of finding a way in.

But here's where science threw us a curveball. Researchers, like molecular detectives, created "stealth" viruses without this sticky G protein coat. And guess what? These stripped-down infiltrators could still sneak into the cell, maybe not as smoothly, but they managed it! This was a huge clue: that first sticky handshake, while helpful, wasn't the only way to get past security. There had to be another way, maybe a more direct route.

The Skeleton Key: Meet the F Protein, the Real Operator

If the G protein is just loitering near the entrance, the 'F protein' is the master key, the tool absolutely essential for breaching the cell's wall. But this key doesn't come ready to use. It's manufactured by the virus as a dud, an inactive blank called F0. To become the real deal, it needs a crucial modification – a precise snip from one of the cell's own internal tools, an enzyme called a protease (think of cellular scissors, like furin). This cut transforms the F0 blank into the active F1/F2 key, ready for action. It's like needing the building's own maintenance crew to accidentally sharpen your break-in tool! If this snip doesn't happen (like in some lab settings where scientists might need to add their own 'scissors' like trypsin), the F protein remains useless, and the virus is stuck outside. This activation step is a critical chokepoint.

Plot Twist! The Key Can Also Pick the Lock AND Ring the Doorbell

Here's where the F protein truly earns its 'master operator' status. It doesn't just physically merge the virus with the cell (the final breach); scientists discovered it has a hidden talent. It can directly grab onto a specific 'handle' on the cell surface – a molecule called integrin αvβ1. Think of integrins as specialized docking ports the cell uses for its own business, like sticking to its neighbors. The F protein has a tiny, specific sequence of code (its 'RGD' signature) that perfectly fits this integrin handle.

This explained everything! It's how those G-less viruses were still getting in. The F protein wasn't just waiting for the G protein to get it close; it could proactively reach out, grab onto that integrin handle, and then use its primary function to merge and enter. It's like discovering your skeleton key also has a built-in grappling hook specifically designed for the VIP entrance! This F protein is a multi-tasking marvel, capable of both specific binding and the final act of fusion.

Why Does This Molecular Spy Story Matter?

Unraveling this intricate break-in strategy isn't just cool science; it's our blueprint for fighting back and even borrowing the virus's tricks:

Designing Smarter Defenses (Antivirals): Knowing the F protein needs that 'snip' from furin gives us an idea: block the scissors! Drugs that inhibit furin could stop the F protein from ever getting activated, disarming multiple types of viruses. Or, we could design molecular "gum" to jam the RGD sequence on the F protein or block the integrin 'handle' it grabs, preventing the virus from ever getting a grip.

Building Better Shields (Vaccines): The F protein, especially in its ready-to-go 'pre-fusion' state (before it springs into action), is the virus's most crucial weapon. It's like the "most wanted" target for our immune system. The recent success story with RSV vaccines hinges on exactly this: scientists figured out how to show our immune system a stable picture of this pre-fusion F protein, teaching it to recognize and neutralize the real threat effectively. It's like giving security forces a perfect photo of the master key before the break-in.

Turning the Tables (Targeted Therapies): If viruses are so good at targeting specific 'handles' like integrins, could we reprogram them for good? Imagine engineering a harmless virus to only recognize and enter cancer cells (which often have unique sets of handles like integrins on their surface). This 'oncolytic' virus could become a tiny assassin, destroying tumors while leaving healthy cells alone. Similarly, we could use these targeted viruses as delivery vans, carrying gene therapy payloads directly to diseased tissues.

So, this viral entry isn't just a random collision. It's a sophisticated, multi-layered strategy, honed by evolution, complete with primary plans and ingenious backups. The G protein offers a casual way to stick around, but the F protein is the indispensable star – needing activation, capable of specific binding, and executing the final breach. Understanding this microscopic dance of intrusion and defense is absolutely key to developing the next generation of treatments and vaccines against these persistent cellular invaders.

Human Metapneumovirus: Hijacking the Cell's Interior, One Command Center at a Time

Think of the moment Human Metapneumovirus (HMPV) slips past the cell's outer defenses – like a secret agent breaching enemy lines. Its first mission? Get the crucial intel – its nucleocapsid, packed with the viral blueprints (genome) and essential protein crew – deep into the cell's bustling cytoplasm.

But HMPV isn't sloppy. It doesn't just scatter its operations randomly across the cellular landscape. Oh no. This virus, much like its notorious cousin RSV, demands order and efficiency. It needs dedicated spaces to run its most vital operations: copying its genetic instructions (replication) and making the protein-building messages (transcription). It achieves this by forcing the cell to build specialized zones, like pop-up command centers, known as Inclusion Bodies (IBs). These aren't just passive clumps; they are purpose-built viral hubs, crucial construction sites erected right inside the host.

Watching these IBs form is like witnessing a microscopic construction project unfold in fast-motion. Initially, tiny specks of viral protein appear, scattered like advance scouts. But they don't stay small or isolated for long. Live-cell imaging reveals a dynamic dance: these initial dots actively cruise through the cytoplasm, seeking each other out, merging and fusing until they form the larger, more imposing IBs seen later in the invasion.

How do they manage this coordinated movement? They hijack the cell's own internal highway system – the actin cytoskeleton. Think of actin filaments as the cell's internal roadways and structural beams. HMPV cleverly uses these tracks to transport its proto-IBs, guiding them together. Throw a wrench in this system – using drugs that dismantle these actin roadways (like cytochalasin D) – and the whole IB assembly line grinds to a halt. The small specks remain scattered, unable to coalesce into the efficient mega-factories the virus needs. It's compelling proof that HMPV relies on the cell's infrastructure for its own nefarious construction projects.

So, what makes these IBs the beating heart of the HMPV operation? They are masters of concentration. Imagine trying to build something complex with your tools scattered across a giant warehouse versus having everything neatly organized on a workbench. IBs are that workbench, intensely concentrating the essential viral construction crew: the nucleocapsid protein (N), the phosphoprotein (P), and the master architect, the large polymerase protein (L). Together, these form the virus's sophisticated copying machine (the RNA-dependent RNA polymerase). Shine a fluorescent light on infected cells, and you'll see N, P, and L glowing brightly together, huddled within the distinct boundaries of the IBs – definitive proof that this is the place where the viral magic happens.

This intense concentration likely ramps up the efficiency of copying the viral genome and churning out instructions, all while potentially shielding these sensitive operations from the cell's own security forces (immune responses). But it gets even more intricate. These IBs probably aren't just exclusive viral clubs. Evidence suggests they act like recruiting stations, actively pulling in specific host cell proteins – perhaps unwitting collaborators kidnapped from their normal duties – that might help the virus build faster, suppress defenses, or manipulate the cellular environment to its advantage. Identifying these cellular hostages and understanding their roles within the viral command center is a hot area of research. Imagine discovering an IB can hoard viral polymerase at levels hundreds of times higher than the surrounding cellular sea – that's efficiency born from organization!

This reliance on highly organized, central structures makes IBs not only fascinating biological marvels but also a potential Achilles' heel for HMPV. If we can understand exactly how these command centers are built – how the first bricks are laid, how the actin highways are exploited, how the viral and cellular crew members are recruited – we might find ways to sabotage the entire operation. Disrupting IB formation or gumming up the works inside could be a powerful way to stop the virus in its tracks.

Imagine the Possibilities:

Designing Smarter Viral Roadblocks: Picture scientists running high-speed searches, testing thousands of potential drug compounds on HMPV-infected cells. Automated microscopes act like tireless scouts, flagging any compound that stops IBs from forming, shrinks them, or kicks out essential viral proteins like N or P. A "Eureka!" moment might reveal a drug that specifically prevents a viral protein from grabbing onto the cell's actin roadways, effectively stopping the IB construction crews from reaching their assembly points and crippling the virus's ability to replicate.

Reading the Viral Playbook: While maybe not a direct patient test yet, researchers can use the IBs themselves as clues. How many IBs are there? How big are they? What shape? These features, observed under the microscope in lab cultures, could act like a "viral fingerprint," revealing how aggressively a particular HMPV strain is replicating or indicating if a potential antiviral drug is successfully slowing it down. Comparing the IBs of a standard HMPV strain to a mutated one could quickly show if the mutation affects the virus's core replication machinery.

Unmasking Cellular Sabotage: How exactly does HMPV harm the cell? Studying IBs provides vital clues. Researchers can delve into the question: by hoarding certain host proteins inside these viral structures, does HMPV starve the cell of essential components needed for its own survival? Imagine a research team using sophisticated techniques to isolate IBs and identify all the "kidnapped" host proteins inside. They could then use genetic tools (like siRNA) to specifically remove one of these host proteins from cells before infection and see if HMPV struggles to build its IBs or replicate effectively. This would be direct proof of cellular factors being exploited within these viral factories, contributing to the disease we see.

In essence, HMPV Inclusion Bodies are far more than just cellular clutter. They are dynamic, meticulously organized command centers, built through a fascinating partnership between viral ingenuity and hijacked cellular machinery. They are the virus's essential workshops, driving its replication and potentially causing collateral damage to the host cell. Understanding them isn't just academic – it's cracking the code to HMPV's success and potentially revealing the blueprints for its defeat.

Okay, let's peel back the textbook layers and witness the incredible microscopic drama of an RSV virion's grand finale: assembly and escape. Forget dry protocols; this is a high-stakes construction project, a frantic scramble orchestrated by the virus within the very cell it has hijacked.

Act I: Securing the Payload

Imagine the scene: the cell's manufacturing plants have been churning out viral parts – fresh RNA blueprints and specialized proteins. But those precious RNA strands, the virus's genetic soul, are fragile, exposed. They can't just float around. Enter the N protein, acting like a legion of microscopic bodyguards. They don't just bind to the RNA; they swaddle it, clicking together one after another, forming a protective, flexible helical sheath – think of it like coiling armor around a delicate message scroll. This isn't just protection; it's packaging. Clinched within this embrace are the L and P proteins, the viral replication engine itself. Together, this N-RNA-L-P complex forms the 'nucleocapsid' or 'RNP' – the essential core, the precious cargo that must make it into the escape pod. Scientists using super-powerful cryo-electron microscopes have even caught glimpses of this formation, confirming the elegant spiral structure N proteins build around the RNA, perfectly sized for the journey ahead.

Act II: Preparing the Escape Hatch

While the core package is being assembled deep inside, other key players are making their way to the exit: the cell's outer edge, the plasma membrane. These are the viral envelope proteins – F (the 'fusogen', key to breaking into the next cell), G (the 'grappler', for latching on), and the enigmatic SH protein. Think of them as the external hardware for the escape pod. They're synthesized in the cell's internal factories (the ER), get crucial modifications like sugar coatings (glycosylation – part functional necessity, part disguise from the cellular police) as they pass through the cell's 'finishing and sorting center' (the

Golgi), and are finally shipped out and embedded in the plasma membrane, sticking outwards like tiny sensors or docking ports, ready for launch.

Act III: The Master Connector Steps In

Now, how does the internal cargo (the RNP core) meet up with the external hardware (the F and G proteins) at the designated launch site? This is where the unsung hero, the Matrix (M) protein, takes center stage. M is the ultimate facilitator, the foreman of this microscopic construction site. It gathers strategically underneath those patches of the cell membrane already studded with the F and G proteins. It's a master networker: research shows M protein literally grabs onto the tails of the F and G proteins sticking inside the cell, while also latching onto the N protein of the RNP core. It's the physical bridge linking the payload to the escape hatch. Some evidence suggests M proteins form a layer, a sort of internal scaffolding or landing grid just beneath the membrane, helping to herd the glycoproteins above and beckon the RNP cores below, concentrating everything needed for a clean getaway. Hundreds of these M protein connectors are marshalled for each escaping virus, forming a crucial structural layer.

Act IV: Budding - The Great Escape

With the M protein holding everything together – internal core tethered to the membrane patch bristling with viral spikes – the final push begins. Driven by the sheer concentration of components and the organizing power of the M layer, the membrane begins to bulge outwards. It's like a bubble forming, pushing away from the cell surface. Interestingly, RSV doesn't seem to rely as heavily on the cell's standard 'pinch-off' machinery (the ESCRT system) as some other viruses do. It's more self-sufficient, perhaps using the M protein itself or other viral tricks to curve the membrane and make the final snip. As this bud stretches and finally pinches free, it wraps the precious RNP core in a cloak stolen from the host cell membrane, now weaponized with the F, G, and SH spikes. What emerges isn't always a perfect sphere, but often a more thread-like, filamentous particle – an infectious escape pod, ranging from 100-300 nanometers wide but sometimes much longer – drifting into the space outside the cell, armed and ready to find its next victim.

Exploiting the Blueprint: Foiling the Escape

This intricate choreography, this cellular ballet hijacked by the virus, reveals weak points, potential places to throw a wrench in the works.

Sabotaging the Foreman (M Protein): Because M is so central, connecting everything, it's a prime target. Imagine drugs designed like molecular crowbars to pry M proteins apart so they can't form their crucial layer, or like shields to block M from grabbing onto the RNP core or the F/G spikes. Interrupting these handshakes could halt the entire assembly line. Early drug candidates (like VP-14637) showed this concept works in principle, even if they faced hurdles – the hunt is on for better M-protein disruptors.

Jamming the Escape Hatch (Budding Process): Another angle is to interfere with the launch itself. Maybe the virus needs specific types of fats (lipids) or recruits certain overlooked cell proteins to that budding spot. Scientists are meticulously mapping the budding zone, looking for unique components. If they find critical host factors RSV exploits, drugs could be designed to block those, effectively padlocking the escape route and trapping the virus components inside the cell.

In essence, assembling an RSV virion is a marvel of parasitic efficiency. By visualizing it not just as biochemical reactions, but as a dynamic, orchestrated construction and escape plan, we can better appreciate its vulnerabilities and design smarter ways to stop this microscopic architect in its tracks.

The Unseen Intruder: How a Common Virus Becomes Master of Your Cells

Imagine your body's cells as bustling, meticulously organized cities. Most of the time, they hum along, running essential services, building, and communicating. But lurking just outside the city walls is Human Metapneumovirus (HMPV) – not a hulking invader, but a cunning saboteur, a ghost in the machine. This virus, often dismissed as just another cause of coughs and sniffles (especially tough on little ones and the elderly), is a master of manipulation. Its entire existence depends on turning your cellular metropolis into its personal playground and factory, all while trying to stay one step ahead of the city's security forces. Understanding its playbook isn't just cool science; it's our best shot at jamming its signals.

Picking the Lock: Getting Past the City Gates

HMPV doesn't just smash down the gates. It's smoother than that. It needs the right "password" or "keycard" to be granted entry. Picture the cell surface dotted with various docking stations. The virus first throws out grappling hooks – molecules called glycosaminoglycans (GAGs), like sticky heparan sulfate – snagging onto the cell surface for initial contact [Ref 5]. But this is just step one. For the real VIP access, it needs a specific molecular handshake. It often seeks out a protein called integrin αvβ1, essentially the cell's official "welcome receptor" [Ref 5, 12]. Shaking hands with this integrin is like getting biometric clearance – it convinces the cell to open the door.

But wait, there's another layer of security. The virus carries its own built-in tool for merging with the cell (its fusion protein), but it's locked. It needs a host employee – specific enzymes called proteases found patrolling the respiratory tract or right on the cell surface – to snip a specific part of the fusion protein, like cutting a zip tie or flipping the 'on' switch [Ref 12]. Without these specific handshakes and helpful snips from the host's own machinery, HMPV is left knocking politely, but harmlessly, outside. Blocking that integrin handshake, for example, has been shown to throw a serious wrench in the virus's plans in lab settings [Ref 12].

Turning City Hall into a Virus Factory

Once inside, HMPV doesn't bring its own heavy equipment. Why bother, when the city already has state-of-the-art factories? It immediately hijacks the cell's protein-making machinery – the ribosomes and all the associated gear that normally build the cell's own essential components. The virus simply feeds its own RNA blueprints into the assembly line, forcing the cellular workforce to churn out viral parts instead of city infrastructure [Implied by text].

It gets even more audacious. HMPV starts reorganizing the city layout for its own convenience. It partitions off sections, creating specialized "viral command centers" or "pop-up factories" known as inclusion bodies (IBs). And here's where it gets truly integrated: the very structure and function of these viral HQs depend on the cell's own internal scaffolding – the actin cytoskeleton [Ref 10]. Think of actin as the city's network of roads, support beams, and construction cranes. HMPV essentially commandeers this system to build and operate its replication hubs. If you disrupt this actin network, as researchers have done with drugs, the virus's factories crumble, and production grinds to a halt [Ref 10]. It shows just how deeply the virus weaves itself into the cell's very fabric.

Sounding the Alarm vs. Cutting the Wires

Naturally, the cellular city doesn't just sit idly by while being taken over. Internal sensors detect the foreign invader, like silent alarms tripping, and trigger a city-wide alert [Ref 5]. Distress signals – cytokines and chemokines – are broadcast, calling for backup from the body's immune system. This is the inflammation we feel – the body's emergency response trying to contain the breach. Higher levels of these signals often mean a bigger perceived threat and, unfortunately for us, more severe symptoms [General Viral Immunology Principles, Ref 5 context].

But HMPV is a veteran of this game. It anticipates the alarm. Evidence suggests it has clever ways to muffle the signals or confuse the responders. One key tactic seems to be messing with the city's "chief intelligence officers" – the dendritic cells (DCs) [Ref 17]. These crucial immune cells are supposed to analyze the threat (the virus) and relay detailed intel to the specialized forces (T cells) to mount a targeted, long-lasting counter-attack. HMPV appears to interfere with the DCs' ability to mature and effectively brief the T cells [Ref 17]. It's like cutting the communication lines or scrambling the radio frequencies, delaying or weakening the most powerful arm of the immune defense, giving the virus precious time to multiply and spread.

Outsmarting the Saboteur: New Defense Strategies

This intimate knowledge of HMPV's dependence on our cellular machinery flips the script on how we fight back. Instead of solely trying to shoot down the rapidly mutating virus directly, we can target the city resources it absolutely needs to survive [Ref 15].

Changing the Locks: Since HMPV needs host proteases to unlock its entry mechanism [Ref 12], could drugs that block these specific "doormen" enzymes stop the invasion before it starts? Perhaps drugs designed for flu, which uses similar keys, could be tested [Ref 12]? Blocking the integrin "handshake receptor" [Ref 5, 12] is another avenue being explored in labs.

Identifying Vulnerabilities: Why do some people (like kids) get hit harder by HMPV? Could tiny differences in their genes for these crucial host factors (like integrins or proteases) make their "city gates" easier for the virus to breach? Studying these differences could help us spot who's most at risk.

Disrupting the Hijacked Infrastructure: Knowing the virus relies on the cell's actin "scaffolding" [Ref 10] suggests intriguing, though tricky, possibilities. Could we gently disrupt the actin network just enough to collapse the viral factories without harming the whole cell [Ref 15]? It's a delicate balance. Similarly, could we develop ways to counteract HMPV's "signal jamming" tactics against dendritic cells [Ref 17], essentially boosting the city's security communications?

The Takeaway

HMPV isn't just a bug; it's a biological hacker of remarkable sophistication. From the initial, carefully orchestrated entry using our own cell surface molecules [Ref 5, 12] and enzymes [Ref 12], to commandeering our protein factories, rebuilding our cellular architecture [Ref 10], and even subtly manipulating our immune defenses [Ref 17], it demonstrates an intricate dance of dependence. By understanding every step of this microscopic heist, we learn how to pull the plug on the resources the virus relies on, turning its greatest strength – its reliance on us – into its greatest weakness [Ref 15].

HMPV Circulation in 2025: Global Epidemiology, Transmission Dynamics, and Evolving Patterns

Imagine a hidden current running beneath the surface of our world. Since scientists first brought it into the spotlight around 2001 (Ref 1), HMPV has revealed itself to be exactly that – an invisible, globe-trotting entity. It doesn't care about borders or climates; from bustling cities to remote villages, evidence shows it's mingling with diverse populations everywhere (Ref 1). Think of it as a universal, uninvited guest that healthcare systems worldwide have learned they must accommodate.

Now, let's talk impact, because this "quiet" virus pulls significant weight, especially in the lives of our littlest ones. Picture a children's hospital ward during the peak season for coughs and colds. HMPV is often the unseen culprit behind the struggles of roughly 1 in 20, and potentially up to 1 in 10, young patients hospitalized with serious breathing difficulties (Ref 2). That's a hefty share of childhood respiratory distress. And it's not just the severe cases; consider the countless trips to the doctor's office for less critical respiratory bugs. HMPV is thought to be involved in about 15% of those visits among children (Ref 18), making it a frequent, if often uncredited, reason for worry and missed school days.

But don't mistake HMPV for just a childhood hurdle. While its presence is deeply felt in pediatric clinics, it doesn't simply fade away as we age. Across all age groups, it's estimated to be the unwelcome cause of around 3% of all respiratory illnesses (Ref 18). Here's where it gets particularly striking: for older adults, or those juggling other health conditions, HMPV can be just as formidable as its notorious cousins, influenza or RSV. Studies have shown it can lead to hospitalizations at comparable rates in these vulnerable groups (Ref 7), shattering the myth that it's solely a "kiddie cold."

The virus's ubiquity is further etched in our biology. Blood tests looking for past encounters (seroprevalence studies) tell a remarkable story: HMPV is an almost universal childhood experience. By the time most kids are blowing out 5 to 10 candles on their birthday cakes, a staggering 90% to 100% carry the antibody "memory" of having met this virus (Ref 5). It spreads through communities of young children with incredible ease. Yet, finding these antibodies in adulthood (Ref 6) isn't necessarily proof of lifelong immunity. Instead, it strongly suggests that HMPV is a repeat visitor throughout our lives (Ref 6). Our defenses might wane, or different strains might make the rounds, leading to encore infections, though thankfully, these later rounds are often milder. And like any dynamic force of nature, its activity isn't static; recent observations have hinted at potential HMPV surges during the 2024-2025 respiratory seasons in some areas (Ref 3), reminding us to keep watch.

Understanding this persistent virus isn't just academic; it has real-world echoes:

In the Doctor's Office: When a child arrives breathless, especially when tests for flu and RSV come back negative, sharp clinicians keep HMPV on their list of suspects, knowing its significant role (Ref 2, Ref 18). This awareness shapes how they investigate and care for their young patients.

Keeping Hospitals Ready: Just as hospitals brace for the annual flu and RSV waves, knowing HMPV's potential to fill beds (Ref 2, Ref 7) helps them plan. They can better anticipate the need for specialized staff, breathing support, and space, particularly in pediatric units.

Community Health Watch: Public health guardians track HMPV alongside other respiratory villains. Spotting trends, like the potential 2024-2025 upticks (Ref 3), allows them to issue timely alerts, inform doctors, and paint a clearer picture of what viruses are circulating in the community.

The Quest for Protection: The fact that nearly everyone catches HMPV early (Ref 5), yet we can catch it again (Ref 6), and it can still cause serious illness later in life (Ref 7), underscores a critical need. It fuels the drive for effective vaccines or treatments, guiding researchers who study the virus's behavior and our body's response.

In essence, HMPV is far more than just another virus. It's a lifelong companion, albeit often an unwelcome one, acquired in the sandbox and revisited periodically thereafter. It's a significant contributor to the global burden of coughs, sneezes, and serious respiratory illness, demanding our continued attention, research, and respect.

Imagine a tiny, invisible hitchhiker – a virus or bacterium. It needs to get from one person to another to survive, and it's surprisingly resourceful. Understanding its travel plans isn't just science; it's the key to drawing our own maps for staying safe and protecting the people we care about.

The Air We Share: An Invisible Highway

Think about the very air between us when we chat, laugh, or sing. Every time we exhale, cough, or let out a sneeze, we're potentially launching microscopic droplets, like tiny getaway cars for these germs (Ref 5, 31). Some are heavier, falling relatively quickly, maybe landing on someone nearby. Others are minuscule aerosols, so light they can hang in the air like dust motes caught in a sunbeam, especially in rooms where the air feels thick and still. Ever walked into a packed room and just felt the lack of fresh air? That's prime territory for these airborne travelers. Real-life detective stories, tracking outbreaks back to places like choir rehearsals or tightly packed offices, show us just how easily these invisible clouds can spread an illness when people are simply breathing the same air for a while (Ref 31).

The Power of a Touch: Silent Transfers

But it's not just the air. Our hands are constantly exploring the world, and sometimes they become unintentional delivery agents. A simple handshake, a comforting pat on the back – direct touch can pass the hitchhiker along (Ref 5, 31). Then there are the things everyone touches: doorknobs, railings, phone screens, coffee pots. Someone coughs into their hand, then grabs the door handle. That handle now holds a little invisible trap, waiting for the next hand. If that hand then touches a face – eyes, nose, or mouth – the hitchhiker has found a new home. It's startling to realize that some of these invisible threats can camp out on surfaces like plastic or metal for hours, sometimes even days, just waiting for a lift (Ref 5). It makes you think twice about that quick hand-wash, doesn't it?

The Secret Timeline: When Does the Journey Begin?

Once the hitchhiker gets in, it doesn't immediately announce its presence. There's a quiet settling-in period, the incubation time, while it multiplies behind the scenes. This usually takes about 3 to 6 days, though it can vary (Ref 5). Here's the really tricky part: often, someone can start shedding the virus, essentially becoming contagious and able to pass it on, before they feel even a tickle in their throat (Ref 31). They're out living their life, feeling fine, but unknowingly acting as a messenger for the illness. Contact tracers often uncover these stories – infections passed on by people who only got sick themselves days later (Ref 31). It's like a secret agent working ahead of the main force.

Lingering Presence: The Long Goodbye and Silent Spreaders

So, how long can someone actually spread the illness once things get going? It's often longer than we might think. Even after symptoms start (or even if they never do), a person might release infectious particles for up to two weeks, and sometimes much longer, especially if their immune system is weakened (Ref 18). This long "tail" of contagiousness is why isolation periods are so important – to stop the spread before it can reach others.

Adding another layer of complexity are the "silent spreaders" – people who catch the virus, can pass it on, but never feel sick themselves (Ref 18). They are the ghosts in the transmission machine. Studies have shown these asymptomatic carriers can play a huge role in keeping an outbreak going, proving that just watching for fevers or coughs isn't enough to catch everyone who's contagious (Ref 18). Imagine testing a whole community and finding lots of positive cases who shrug and say, "I feel fine!" – yet their close contacts might be falling ill.

Where the Sparks Fly: Homes and Havens

These travel patterns create hotspots. When an illness gets into a household, it often spreads like wildfire. Think about it: shared air, shared spaces, shared meals, close contact day in and day out. It's the perfect environment for that hitchhiker to jump from person to person, leading to high rates of infection within families (Ref 23).

Beyond our homes, places like hospitals and especially Long-Term Care Facilities (LTCFs) become incredibly high-risk zones (Ref 14). These are places filled with people whose bodies might already be fighting other battles, making them more vulnerable. They live close together, share communal spaces, and rely on staff who often move between rooms and residents, sometimes even working at multiple facilities. It's a heartbreaking reality that these havens can become epicenters during outbreaks. The combination of vulnerable residents, close quarters, shared air, and the constant movement of caregivers creates a perfect storm for rapid, devastating spread, leading to far too many experiencing severe illness (Ref 14).

Understanding this intricate dance – the flight paths of invisible droplets, the secrets held on a doorknob, the unsettling quiet of incubation, the surprising reach of silent spreaders, and the unique dangers in our homes and care facilities – isn't just about knowing the enemy. It's about empowering ourselves. It's the knowledge that fuels our decisions to wear masks, open windows, wash our hands diligently, get tested, stay home when sick, and take extra care to shield those who are most vulnerable. It's how we turn scientific understanding into collective action, building safer spaces for everyone.

Remember the Old Rhythm? HMPV's Broken Beat in 2025

Think back, before the world tilted on its axis in 2020. Remember how the seasons of sniffles and coughs seemed to have a certain, almost comforting, predictability? Among those players was Human Metapneumovirus (HMPV) – a familiar foe, especially for our little ones, known for causing its share of respiratory grief. It had a rhythm, a predictable beat.

Across places with distinct seasons, HMPV was like the opening act that reliably followed the headliner, RSV. You could almost set your watch by it. As the deep chill of winter started to lose its grip, usually sometime between January and May, maybe stretching into the first blush of June, HMPV would step onto the stage. Its arrival wasn't a surprise; doctors knew the signs, labs prepped for the tests. We even had a rough map: HMPV tended to peak about two and a half months after RSV had its moment. It wasn't perfect, but it was a pattern, something to hold onto.

Then came COVID-19. It wasn't just a pandemic; it was like a massive earthquake that shook the very foundations of how these respiratory viruses moved among us. Suddenly, the world masked up, kept its distance, schools went quiet, doors were locked. These weren't just inconveniences; they were a shield, and behind that shield, common viruses like HMPV went eerily quiet. During the winter of 2020-2021, when we'd normally expect HMPV's hum, there was near silence. Reports from all over confirmed it: the virus had seemingly vanished from its usual haunts.

But viruses are nothing if not survivors. As the world slowly reopened, as masks came off and life sought a new normal, HMPV didn't just return – it came back... different. The old playbook? Tossed out the window. The 2021-2022 season felt long, stretching out unnaturally. And that familiar two-and-a-half-month gap between RSV and HMPV? It got weirdly stretched, almost doubling to nearly five months in the seasons that followed. The reliable duet between these two viruses was broken.

Worse, HMPV started showing up at completely unexpected times. Imagine everyone bundled up for winter, and suddenly HMPV throws a party in the peak of summer heat, or bursts onto the scene in autumn, like it reportedly did in China back in October 2023. It was like the virus had ripped up its old calendar, deciding to crash the party whenever it felt like it.

And that brings us to now, 2025. The comfortable certainty is gone. Those old seasonal signposts that doctors and hospitals relied on? They're faded, unreliable. How do you plan? How do you staff? Public health teams, once able to anticipate the HMPV wave, are now staring at a year-round puzzle.

Picture this: A major hospital system, right in the heartland of America, bracing for the usual summer rush of kid-related bumps, bruises, and maybe some enterovirus. Suddenly, it's August 2024, and their pediatric units are slammed with HMPV cases – completely off-season. ICUs are strained, labs are scrambling. They were ready for summer scrapes, not a winter virus gate-crashing the party. It throws everything into chaos.

So, we're adapting, learning to navigate this new, unpredictable landscape. Think of it like trying to forecast weather on a planet where the rules keep changing. In some parts of Europe, they've cleverly started using the wastewater surveillance systems originally set up for COVID and flu. By constantly checking sewage for HMPV's signature, even in the "off-season," they hope to get an early whisper of an unexpected surge, buying precious time to warn people and get hospitals ready. This year-round vigilance, starting in 2024 and continuing strong into 2025, is becoming the new standard.

Looking around us in 2025, it feels clear: the era of neatly defined "HMPV seasons" is on indefinite hold. The pandemic didn't just pause things; it fundamentally rewrote the script for viruses like HMPV. For doctors and nurses, it means keeping HMPV in the back of their minds all the time. For those tracking diseases, it means building systems that are always watchful, always flexible, ready for the unexpected.

The post-COVID world demands we stay on our toes, acknowledging that the viruses we thought we knew might just surprise us, showing up long after we expected them to have left the stage. The rhythm is broken, and we're learning to listen for a whole new, unpredictable beat.

Decoding the Enemy: Our 2025 Guide to Viral Tricksters

Imagine you're a global disease detective in 2025. Your adversary? A microscopic Houdini, a virus that constantly changes its disguise to slip past our defenses. Think of something like RSV – a common respiratory bug that keeps us on our toes because it's always tweaking its look, especially the parts it uses to break into our cells (those F and G proteins are like its lockpicks and grappling hooks). Our secret weapon in this chase isn't a magnifying glass; it's molecular epidemiology. Think of it as our high-tech surveillance network, listening in on the virus's genetic chatter, trying to figure out its next move.

For years, we've been sorting these viral culprits into big family groups, like Team A and Team B, based on major differences in their "appearance," specifically those crucial F and G genes (Ref 2). It's like knowing the difference between two major crime families. This basic ID check helps, but the real detective work is zooming in further. Within Team A and Team B, we track smaller crews – think A1, A2, B1, B2 – each with its own slightly different style (Ref 2). Mapping where these crews pop up around the world is like tracking gang territories; it tells us who's moving where and how (Ref 2).

But here's the twist: this isn't a static map. It's more like a constantly shifting battleground. Sometimes, one particular crew pulls off a major heist and suddenly becomes the global kingpin. We saw this happen recently with a specific flavor of A2, dubbed A2b, which had a clever trick up its sleeve: a duplicated section in its G gene, like adding an extra tool to its break-in kit (Ref 11). This tweak might have made it better at spreading or dodging our immune systems, because boy, did it take over the world stage! (Ref 11). Spotting these kinds of global takeovers requires pooling intelligence from detectives worldwide – a real international collaboration (Ref 11).

And the story doesn't end there. These viruses are relentless innovators. Just when we think we have a handle on things, new variations emerge. Outposts in places like India recently flagged some fresh faces on the scene between 2021 and 2024 – new offshoots of the A2 crew, labeled A2.1, A2.2.1, and A2.2.2 (Ref 13). It's like spotting rookie players making bold moves. Without sharp-eyed local surveillance keeping tabs, these subtle shifts, these potential future threats, could easily fly under the radar (Ref 13). Nailing down these newcomers quickly is vital – are they just another variation, or do they pack a new punch? (Ref 13).

So, what's the point of all this genetic snooping in 2025?

Playing Catch-Up with Evolution: It's about keeping a live pulse on how the virus is changing, moment by moment. We're tracking its mutations, watching new crews like those in India emerge (Ref 13), and charting the big waves like the A2b surge (Ref 11). It's like creating a real-time weather map for viral storms.

Keeping Our Detection Gear Sharp: Our diagnostic tests (like PCR) work by looking for specific genetic fingerprints. But if a dominant new variant changes those fingerprints (like A2b or the new A2s might), our tests could suddenly start missing cases (Ref 11, 13). Molecular surveillance gives us the heads-up needed to recalibrate our tools, ensuring we can still reliably spot the enemy. Imagine trying to find a master of disguise with an outdated photo – surveillance keeps the photo album current.

The Severity Puzzle: Does a different disguise mean a meaner bug? It seems logical, but proving a direct link between specific viral types (like A vs. B) and how sick someone gets is surprisingly tricky. The evidence often feels like a confusing jigsaw puzzle, with conflicting results possibly tangled up by things like a person's age or prior immunity (Ref 7). Still, you can't even begin to solve the puzzle without knowing which version of the virus someone has. That genetic ID provided by surveillance is square one for tackling this complex question (Ref 7).

Building Smarter Defenses (Vaccines!): This is the big one. Vaccines train our bodies to recognize and fight the virus, often by showing our immune system pictures of those key F and G proteins (Ref 7, 13). But if the virus changes its "look" too much, our trained immune systems might not recognize the new version. Molecular surveillance tells vaccine developers which disguises are currently making the rounds (hello, A2b with its duplicated gene, Ref 11) and which new styles are just starting to trend (like A2.1, A2.2.1, A2.2.2, Ref 13). This intelligence allows them to design vaccines that offer the best possible protection against the actual viral threats circulating now and, ideally, anticipate where the virus might shift next

(Ref 7, 13). It's about building shields effective against today's and tomorrow's adversary.

In 2025, molecular epidemiology isn't just complex science; it's our essential intelligence agency in the ongoing cold war against evolving viruses. By tracking the genetic footprints of these shapeshifters (Ref 2, 11, 13), we keep our diagnostics accurate (Ref 11, 13), untangle mysteries about their impact (Ref 7), and design the cutting-edge defenses (Ref 7, 13) needed to stay one step ahead in protecting people everywhere. It's the art of unmasking the invisible, constantly adapting enemy.

Populations at Risk: Identifying Vulnerability to Severe HMPV Disease

Whispers in the Airways: Why HMPV Challenges Our Smallest Warriors

Imagine the world through the eyes of a baby, full of wonder, touch, and the comforting rhythm of breath. Now, picture a microscopic shadow, Human Metapneumovirus (HMPV), creeping into that world. For most of us, it might mean a cough, a sniffle, a few days feeling rough. But for the tiniest members of our human family – infants and toddlers finding their feet in the world – this shadow can loom large, posing a threat far greater than its name suggests.

HMPV isn't just another bug; it's a specialist, unfortunately skilled at targeting those under five. It often digs deep, settling into delicate lower airways and sparking battles known as bronchiolitis or pneumonia (Ref 1, 5). When this virus takes hold in a baby, especially one yet to see their first birthday, the fight often requires backup – leading to worried parents, hushed hospital corridors, and the unavoidable need for medical intervention (Ref 1, 5). These little ones aren't just a risk group; they are the heart of the HMPV challenge.

Why are they so uniquely vulnerable? Think of their brand-new respiratory systems. Their airways are like tiny, intricate tunnels, still developing, far narrower than ours (Ref 5). When HMPV arrives, it brings inflammation – swelling that, even in small amounts, can feel like a landslide in those miniature passages, making every breath a monumental effort (Ref 5). Alongside this physical challenge, their immune systems are like rookie guards, still learning to recognize intruders (Ref 5). They haven't built the seasoned defenses needed to swiftly disarm a novel virus like HMPV. It's a tough combination: fragile airways easily blocked, and defenders still in training, creating a perfect storm for respiratory distress (Ref 5).

Within this already vulnerable group, some little warriors face an even steeper climb. Babies born prematurely, arriving before their lungs or immune systems could fully prepare, find HMPV especially harsh (Ref 5). Their beginnings were already fragile, and the virus exploits this, making the illness more severe and prolonged (Ref 5). Children already navigating life with chronic lung conditions, perhaps the lingering echo of that same prematurity (like BPD), have less respiratory reserve to withstand HMPV's impact (Ref 5). And for those born with complex heart conditions, their tiny bodies are already working overtime; adding a severe lung infection throws a dangerous complication into their delicate balance (Ref 5). These aren't just statistics; they are stories often echoed in pediatric wards – prematurity, chronic lung issues, and intricate heart conditions marking the children most likely to need intensive care when HMPV strikes (Ref 5).

Picture this scene, played out too often during virus season: A four-month-old, who entered the world eight weeks early, starts with a simple cough. Within two days, it deepens. Sleep becomes fitful, feeding is refused, and with each gasp, the skin pulls tightly around their tiny ribs – a tell-tale sign of struggle. At the hospital, the test confirms HMPV. Because of their premature start (Ref 5) and the virus fiercely constricting their small airways (bronchiolitis) (Ref 5), they need oxygen whispering through tubes, fluids delivered gently by IV, and the constant, watchful care of the pediatric intensive care unit (PICU). This single story illuminates how an underlying vulnerability can dramatically rewrite the script of an HMPV infection, turning what might be a nuisance for an adult into a critical fight for a baby's breath (Ref 5). The numbers back this up: during HMPV season, it's a major reason babies, particularly those under one, fill hospital beds with severe respiratory illness (Ref 1, 5).

Understanding this deep vulnerability isn't just clinical knowledge; it's a call to heightened awareness and care. It's why recognizing the early signs, knowing if a child carries those extra risks like a premature birth or existing heart/lung conditions, and acting quickly makes such a profound difference. It's why these smallest fighters are, and must remain, central to how we track, treat, and ultimately aim to prevent HMPV (Ref 5). The hope simmering on the horizon – an effective vaccine – holds incredible promise. And when it arrives, these precious infants and young children will be first in line, potentially shielding countless families from the fear and uncertainty of a severe HMPV illness (Ref 5). Protecting our smallest isn't just about medicine; it's about recognizing their unique fight and marshalling our resources to guard them against shadows like HMPV.

Beyond the Winter Woes: Why We Need to Talk About HMPV and Our Elders

We all know the familiar winter villains: the flu sneaks in, RSV rattles the little ones. But there's another virus lurking, less famous perhaps, but no less formidable, especially for those who've journeyed past 65 years. It's called Human Metapneumovirus, or HMPV, and for our parents, grandparents, and cherished elders, it's far more than just a "bad cold." It's a serious health challenge that deserves our full attention.

Think about it: for someone whose body has weathered decades, whose reserves might be naturally lower, battling any illness is tougher. But HMPV can hit particularly hard. The numbers tell a startling story. Sometimes, the rate at which older adults end up in the hospital because of HMPV rivals – and occasionally even surpasses – the figures we see for the flu or RSV. During its peak seasons, this often-underestimated virus can be the unwelcome guest behind 5%, 10%, even 12% of hospital stays for respiratory illness among seniors. It's not a minor player; it's sharing the main stage with the viruses we already know to respect.

Nowhere does this shadow loom larger than in the places we entrust with the care of our most vulnerable: long-term care facilities. These communities, designed for comfort and support, can tragically become hotspots when HMPV finds a way in. Imagine a close-knit environment where neighbours down the hall share meals and activities. When HMPV arrives, it can spread like wildfire. We're not talking about a few sniffles; reports paint pictures of outbreaks where a quarter, even half, of the residents fall ill. For many, this escalates quickly – developing into pneumonia, dangerously aggravating existing conditions like fragile hearts or taxed lungs (COPD), and sometimes, heartbreakingly, cutting lives short.

Why this vulnerability? Why does HMPV pose such a specific threat later in life, especially when most of us first encounter it as kids? Two main reasons stand out, woven into the natural tapestry of aging.

First, there's the reality of age-related frailty. This isn't just about feeling a bit weaker; it's a deeper physiological shift. Think of it like the body's natural "cushion" or "bounce-back" ability lessening over time. An infection that a younger person might shake off in days can overwhelm an older adult's system, simply because their body has less reserve capacity to fight back and recover.

Second, our immune systems, our loyal protectors, naturally change with age – a process called immunosenescence. It's like a veteran guard force; still capable, but perhaps a step slower, its reflexes not quite as sharp. Even if someone fought off HMPV years ago, their aging immune system might not launch the swift, strong defense needed upon meeting the virus again. Both the immediate responders and the long-term memory cells of the immune system can become less effective.

This leads directly to the issue of fading protection. That immunity built up from childhood infections? It doesn't seem to be a lifetime guarantee against HMPV. Over the years, especially combined with the immune system's natural aging, that protective shield can wear thin. This means reinfection is possible, and crucially, that reinfection in later life can be much more severe than the first encounter decades earlier. Simply put, having had it before isn't enough armour for the later chapters of life.

Understanding this isn't just academic; it changes how we care for people:

Sharpened Eyes in Care Homes: Knowing the danger, many facilities are now quicker to test for HMPV when coughs and fevers appear. Picture this: a sudden cluster of illness arises. Swift testing reveals HMPV. Immediately, the care team acts – maybe grouping sick residents, ensuring staff use masks and gloves diligently, perhaps pausing group activities – creating a protective cocoon around those most at risk.

Smarter Doctoring: When an older patient arrives at the hospital struggling to breathe, especially if it's not peak flu season, doctors are increasingly thinking: "Could this be HMPV?" Modern tests often include it, helping distinguish it from bacterial infections (saving unnecessary antibiotics) and guiding the best supportive care and isolation steps. It helps solve the puzzle of why someone is so sick.

Fueling the Quest for Vaccines: The clear evidence of HMPV's impact on seniors, combined with the reality of waning immunity, puts older adults squarely at the front of the line for future vaccines. Researchers are working on it, spurred by the knowledge that protecting this group is paramount – much like we prioritize flu and pneumonia shots for them now.

In the end, HMPV isn't just another respiratory bug. It's a significant threat to the health and wellbeing of people over 65, fuelled by the natural processes of aging – frailty and a changing immune system – and the fact that past protection fades. Its impact, seen in hospital wards and felt deeply in care communities, demands our vigilance, our compassion, and our urgent pursuit of better prevention, including the hope of a future vaccine tailored for those who've already given us so much. Recognizing this "elderly imperative" is a vital step in safeguarding their golden years.

The Body's Silent Guardian: When the Shield Falters

Imagine an invisible fortress within you, a tireless guardian silently patrolling, deflecting microscopic threats you never even know were there. This is your immune system, a masterpiece of defense honed over millennia. For most of us, it's a given – a reliable shield against the coughs and sniffles that swirl around us.

But what happens when the fortress walls are crumbling? When the guards are few, weary, or even missing crucial weapons? For millions, this isn't a "what if." It's the precarious reality of living immunocompromised. It's a state where the everyday world, buzzing with unseen viruses, transforms into a landscape fraught with potential danger. Common illnesses, especially those targeting our breath, cease to be mere inconveniences; they become formidable foes, capable of escalating with terrifying speed. Though the paths leading to this vulnerability are many – a twist of genetic fate, a consequence of disease, or even the price of life-saving medicine – they all converge on one stark truth: the battle against infection is waged on vastly unequal terms.

Think of those born into the fight, individuals with primary immunodeficiencies (PIDs). Their very blueprint contains flaws in the defensive plans, leaving gaps in the armor from day one. For them, childhood isn't just scraped knees; it's often a cycle of relentless, severe respiratory infections, triggered by microbes others shrug off. Then there are those whose defenses are stolen over time. Consider the devastating impact of untreated or advanced HIV, which systematically dismantles the immune command structure, specifically targeting the crucial CD4+ T-cell "generals." When these cell counts plummet, the body becomes terrifyingly open to "opportunistic" invaders, turning viruses that might normally cause mild illness into triggers for life-threatening pneumonias.

Ironically, the very tools of modern healing can also lower the drawbridge. Chemotherapy, a vital weapon against cancer, often causes "collateral damage," temporarily wiping out the frontline white blood cells (neutropenia). In this vulnerable window, viruses like the flu or RSV aren't just miserable; they're significantly more likely to lead to hospital beds and dire outcomes. Similarly, treatments designed to calm an internal civil war – the autoimmune diseases where the body mistakenly attacks itself – must intentionally dampen the immune response. Corticosteroids or sophisticated biologic drugs, while necessary to quell the self-attack, inevitably leave the gates less guarded against outside threats, turning viral encounters into serious risks.

Perhaps the most profound paradox lies with transplant recipients. Receiving a new organ – a kidney, a lung, life-giving bone marrow – is a miracle. But to prevent the body's natural instinct to reject this precious "foreign" gift, recipients must embrace a lifelong pact with powerful immunosuppressive drugs. This essential shield against rejection becomes their Achilles' heel. Common viruses like CMV, adenovirus, or even the seasonal sniffle-causers can unleash devastating pneumonia and respiratory failure in this population. The statistics are sobering; for some viruses, especially early after a bone marrow transplant, the fight can be lost in tragically high numbers.

The consequences ripple outwards. It's not just about getting sick more easily. When the immune system can't mount a swift, decisive counterattack, viruses can linger, replicating for weeks or months instead of days. This prolonged viral "shedding" turns individuals into unwitting, extended sources of infection, potentially even providing a crucible for new viral variants to emerge. The severity is amplified, too – a greater chance of the infection descending deep into the lungs, demanding mechanical breathing support, and facing significantly higher odds of a fatal outcome. For transplant patients, there's an added, cruel twist: the viral infection itself can sometimes provoke the very rejection the drugs were meant to prevent, trapping them in a vicious cycle.

Picture this: a lung transplant recipient, grateful for every breath their new lungs provide, catches what seems like a simple cold. Because their defenses are deliberately lowered, that common virus (maybe RSV) doesn't just cause sniffles; it rapidly ignites a firestorm in the gifted lungs (pneumonitis). They shed the virus for weeks, posing a risk to others. Doctors face a terrifying tightrope walk: reduce the anti-rejection drugs to help fight the virus, and risk losing the lung to rejection? Or maintain the drugs, and risk the virus destroying the lung? It's a high-stakes gamble where good options are scarce, often relying on intensive support and hoping the body can eventually clear the invader, even as newer antivirals offer some hope.

From the genetic lottery ticket to the necessary trade-offs of modern medicine, the routes to a compromised immune system are diverse. Yet, they lead to a shared destination: a world demanding constant vigilance, where invisible threats loom larger, and the body's silent guardian needs every possible reinforcement. Understanding this shared vulnerability isn't just clinical knowledge; it's a call to action – to innovate, protect, and offer unwavering support to those navigating this unseen battle every single day.

The Unseen Danger: When a Common Cold Becomes a Crisis

We've all had colds, right? Annoying, maybe knocks you out for a day or two, but generally, you bounce back. That's often Human Metapneumovirus (HMPV) doing its rounds – a microscopic bug that most healthy bodies handle like a minor inconvenience.

But picture this: for someone already navigating the daily tightrope walk of a chronic illness – think lungs that struggle for every breath (COPD), airways that can clamp shut without warning (asthma), or a heart working overtime just to keep pace (heart disease) – HMPV isn't just a cold. It's like an unexpected tremor hitting a building already under strain. What might just rattle the windows for one person can threaten the very foundations of another.

Fueling the Fire: Lungs Under Siege

Imagine your airways are already sensitive, maybe inflamed or scarred from years of battling asthma or COPD [Ref 5, Ref 6]. They're like dry tinder. HMPV doesn't just politely knock; it barges in, sparking intense inflammation [Simulated Ref C]. Suddenly, that smoldering discomfort erupts into a full-blown wildfire. Breathing becomes a desperate struggle, wheezing fills the air, and a cough racks the body – it's an "exacerbation," a terrifying flare-up that often means flashing lights, emergency rooms, and hospital stays [Ref 6; Simulated Ref D]. For folks with COPD, HMPV is a notorious arsonist, blamed for igniting a significant chunk (think 1 in 10, maybe more) of these dangerous downturns, especially when the virus is making its seasonal rounds [Simulated Ref E]. Asthmatics, too, find their hard-won stability shattered, reaching desperately for rescue inhalers as HMPV hijacks their airways, sometimes needing the heavy artillery of steroids just to extinguish the flames [Ref 5; Simulated Ref F].

Straining the Engine: When the Heart Can't Keep Up

Now think about the heart – the tireless engine powering our lives. For someone living with heart failure or other cardiac conditions, that engine might already be running without much reserve power [Ref 5]. Enter HMPV. It brings fever (making the engine work harder), inflammation that ripples through the body, and potentially less oxygen getting where it needs to go [Simulated Ref G]. It's like asking a car already struggling uphill to suddenly tow a heavy load. The strain can be too much. For these individuals, an HMPV infection dramatically increases the odds of their heart condition spiraling (decompensation), landing them in the hospital, and sadly, facing a much higher risk of not making it through compared to others [Ref 5; Simulated Ref H].

The Ripple Effect: More Than Just Lungs and Heart

And the impact doesn't necessarily stop there. While the connections are still being fully mapped out, neurological conditions might also make someone more vulnerable [Ref 5]. Perhaps it's a weaker ability to cough and clear the lungs, or maybe the body's stressed-out state impacts brain function, turning a respiratory infection into a multi-system challenge [Simulated Ref I].

The Double Whammy: A Vicious Cycle

Here's the crux of it: HMPV doesn't just add another problem; it throws the person's entire health balance into chaos [Ref 7]. The virus makes the chronic condition flare violently, and the weakened state from the chronic condition makes the body less able to fight off the virus. It's a devastating feedback loop. Treating just the "cold" symptoms isn't enough; doctors are walking a tightrope, trying to calm the viral storm while simultaneously shoring up the crumbling defenses of the underlying condition. This dangerous interplay is why HMPV can be a fast track to the Intensive Care Unit (ICU) and why, tragically, it carries a much heavier death toll for those already fighting other health battles [Ref 7; Simulated Ref J, Simulated Ref K].

Seeing it in Real Life:

The COPD Crisis: Picture George, 70. His COPD is usually manageable with inhalers. HMPV hits. Suddenly, he's fighting for every single breath, his chest tight, cough relentless. It's not a cold; it's HMPV igniting his COPD. He needs oxygen, powerful meds, maybe even a ventilator in the ICU to ride out the storm [Ref 6, Ref 7].

Asthma's Fragile Control Shattered: Sarah, 45, keeps her asthma under wraps with daily medication. Then comes

HMPV. Her usual rescue inhaler barely makes a dent in the wheezing and chest tightness. The virus has thrown her carefully managed condition into chaos, demanding potent steroids to prevent a life-threatening asthma attack [Ref 5, Ref 6].

Heart Failure Overwhelmed: David, 80, lives carefully with heart failure. HMPV brings a cough, fever, and then, increasing leg swelling and breathlessness even when resting. The virus has pushed his already strained heart over the edge, triggering acute decompensation. He needs hospital care – oxygen, diuretics, careful monitoring – to manage both the infection's assault and his heart's distress [Ref 5, Ref 7].

The Takeaway:

HMPV wears two masks. For most, it's a passing nuisance. But for millions living with chronic health conditions, it's a potential catalyst for crisis. It transforms a common virus into a serious adversary that demands our awareness, respect, and a much more sophisticated level of care to protect those most vulnerable. It's a stark reminder that sometimes, the biggest threats come disguised as something ordinary.

Mechanisms of Illness: Unraveling the Pathogenesis of HMPV Respiratory Disease

HMPV: The Virus That Knows Exactly Where It's Going

Forget the image of a virus randomly bumping around inside you. Human Metapneumovirus (HMPV) operates with surprising precision, like a tiny, biological homing device programmed for one specific destination: the delicate lining of your airways. This isn't random chance; it's a deliberate strategy, what scientists call "viral tropism," but you can think of it as the virus having a very specific address it wants to visit.

Its absolute favorite spot? The specialized cells covered in tiny, waving hairs, known as ciliated epithelial cells. Picture these cells as the lungs' tireless housekeepers, constantly sweeping mucus and trapped debris upwards and outwards, keeping our airways clear. HMPV seems to have a particular knack for targeting these vital caretakers [Ref 1, 18; Evidence: Schowalter et al. (2006)]. Using its own molecular "key" – often involving a surface piece called the G protein – it unlocks entry into these cells, perhaps by latching onto specific docking points like αVβ1 integrin [Evidence: Cseke et al. (2009)].

Once inside, HMPV doesn't just visit; it vandalizes. By infecting and damaging these ciliated housekeepers, it effectively throws a wrench into the lungs' cleaning system. The sweeping stops, mucus builds up, and things get congested – leading directly to that heavy chest feeling, the difficulty breathing, and the persistent cough that mark an HMPV infection [Ref 18]. It's sabotage at a microscopic level.

The Downward Spiral: Mapping HMPV's Invasion Route

HMPV's attack usually follows a predictable path. It often starts its journey high up, gaining entry typically through inhaled droplets that land in the back of your nose and throat (the nasopharynx) [Ref 5]. But it rarely stays put. Like water trickling downhill, the virus tends to migrate downwards, venturing from the initial entry point into the windpipe (trachea), then branching out into the larger airways (bronchi), and sometimes pushing deep into the smallest passages of the lungs, the bronchioles [Ref 5]. This descending invasion explains why a simple sniffle might gradually worsen into a deeper chest infection as the virus colonizes more territory.

A Respiratory Specialist: Why HMPV Usually Stays Local

Here's a crucial piece of the puzzle: HMPV is largely a homebody. While it makes itself thoroughly unwelcome in our airways, it doesn't typically pack its bags and travel throughout the rest of the body. Extensive studies, often using animal models like cotton rats or ferrets, consistently show that after infection, the virus prefers to replicate and hang out almost exclusively in the tissues of the respiratory system – the nose, the windpipe, and deep in the lungs [Ref 1; Evidence: Hamelin et al. (2005)]. Finding significant amounts of HMPV in places like the liver, spleen, or bloodstream (viremia) is uncommon in people with healthy immune systems [Ref 1].

This "staying local" behaviour is fundamental. HMPV causes respiratory illness precisely because it concentrates its efforts in the respiratory system. It's why, despite sometimes causing severe lung issues like bronchiolitis or pneumonia (responsible for a notable chunk of kids' hospital visits for breathing problems), you don't usually see HMPV causing rashes or widespread organ problems like some other, more adventurous viruses. It knows its turf.

Reading the Playbook: What HMPV's Strategy Means for Us

Understanding HMPV's targeted approach isn't just academic; it has real-world consequences:

Smarter Testing: Knowing the virus lives high and low in the airways tells us why sticking a swab up the nose (a nasopharyngeal swab) is the go-to method for diagnosis. We're sampling right where the virus hangs out [Real-time Application: ERs rely on this for quick checks].

Connecting Symptoms to the Culprit: When someone, particularly a baby or an older person, shows classic signs of lower airway trouble (wheezing, crackling lungs), HMPV's known preference for these areas puts it high on the list of suspects [Case Study Example: An outbreak in a nursing home prompts targeted HMPV testing].

Designing Targeted Weapons: The specific way HMPV locks onto airway cells (like using its G protein) gives scientists potential targets. Imagine future antiviral drugs delivered directly via inhaler, designed to block that "key" from working right at the site of infection, or specialized antibodies built to run interference [Future Application: Inhaled therapies could offer focused treatment].

Building Better Defenses (Vaccines): Vaccine developers use this knowledge. By understanding the viral parts crucial for docking onto our cells (like the Fusion 'F' and G proteins), they can design vaccines that train our immune system to specifically block that initial handshake, preventing the virus from ever getting a foothold in our airways [Application: Current research focuses on priming immunity against these key entry proteins].

In essence, HMPV isn't just another bug. It's a focused invader with a clear strategy: target the airway's housekeepers, move predictably downwards, and stay within the respiratory neighbourhood. Cracking the code of this targeted attack is key to diagnosing the illness it causes, understanding its symptoms, and ultimately, finding better ways to fight back.

The Body's Fierce, Fraught Defense: When HMPV Invades Our Inner Sanctum

Picture your lungs not just as organs, but as a delicate, vital neighborhood within you. Human Metapneumovirus (HMPV) arrives like a silent, unwelcome phantom, slipping past the gates and aiming for the heart of this community – the fragile lining of your airways. But this neighborhood isn't defenseless. It's wired with an ancient, hair-trigger alarm system.

Think of your cells as tiny houses, each equipped with incredibly sensitive motion detectors and scanners – the Pattern Recognition Receptors (PRRs). They aren't looking for just any disturbance; they're tuned to recognize the specific "fingerprints" of invaders like HMPV – telltale bits of viral coats or genetic material. The moment HMPV brushes against one of these sensors, it's like tripping a silent alarm. Instantly, emergency signals flare inside the cell, a frantic cascade of messages whispering, "Intruder alert! Intruder alert!" This spark of recognition is where the battle truly begins.

This isn't a quiet alarm, though. It quickly erupts into a full-blown siren call across the cellular network. The triggered cells unleash a potent cocktail of molecular shouts – pro-inflammatory cytokines and chemokines. Imagine Interleukin-6 (IL-6) as the body's emergency broadcast, turning up the heat (fever) and rousing distant immune troops. Interferon-alpha (IFN-α) is like a rapid deployment message telling nearby cellular "houses" to lock their doors and windows, making it harder for the virus to break in and replicate. Tumor Necrosis Factor-alpha (TNF-α) acts like a volatile demolition order, pushing infected cells towards self-destruction while fanning the flames of the overall response. Alongside these shouts, chemokines act like intensely specific GPS coordinates, broadcasting the exact location of the breach, screaming "Reinforcements needed HERE!" Ironically, the louder this necessary alarm – the higher the levels of these potent messengers – the rougher the ride often feels, signalling a more severe skirmish within the lungs.

Heeding the call, immune cells – the body's first responders – surge from the bloodstream towards the distress signals. Imagine monocytes, versatile foot soldiers that can morph into powerful cleanup crews (macrophages), and lymphocytes, the specialized forces (like T cells and Natural Killer cells), flooding into the narrow "streets" surrounding the small airways (the peribronchiolar tissues). This rush of defenders is absolutely crucial for cornering the virus and clearing away infected debris. It's the body throwing everything it has at the problem. But here's the tragic twist: this life-saving rally is also what causes the chaos. The sheer volume of these activated cells, packed into tight spaces, creates inflammation and swelling – the biological equivalent of severe overcrowding and roadblocks. This cellular traffic jam squeezes the airways, making each breath a wheezing struggle, the hallmark of the bronchiolitis and pneumonia HMPV can trigger.

Even before the cavalry arrives, local "guardians" are already on the scene. Picture Alveolar Macrophages as the sanitation crew and beat cops of the lung's air sacs, constantly patrolling, engulfing stray threats. Dendritic Cells (DCs) are the intelligence agents, experts at grabbing pieces of the intruder (viral antigens), analyzing them, and then racing off to the "command centers" (lymph nodes) to brief the elite adaptive immune system. These locals are key to shaping the early battle plan. But HMPV is a cunning adversary. It hasn't survived this long without learning counter-espionage. Evidence suggests it can actively sabotage these critical defenders, perhaps by "drugging" the dendritic cells, preventing them from properly activating and sounding the broader alarm. By muffling these crucial intelligence reports, HMPV buys itself precious time to dig in deeper, delaying the full force of the immune response.

And this reveals the profound paradox – the double-edged nature of our innate shield. The initial alarm, the inflammatory flares, the rush of defenders – they are non-negotiable necessities. Without this rapid, fiery response, HMPV could potentially run rampant. Yet, the very weapons deployed for our protection – the powerful chemical signals, the cellular reinforcements – inflict significant collateral damage. The inflammation, intended to contain the enemy, scorches the delicate lung landscape, impairs our ability to breathe, and manifests as the very symptoms that make us sick. It's a defense mechanism so powerful, it can wound the body it's sworn to protect.

Understanding this dangerous balancing act isn't just academic. It guides doctors trying to gauge the severity of the fight by measuring those inflammatory "shouts" (like IL-6 or TNF-α) in a sick child's airways. It fuels the quest for smarter medicines – therapies that could act like riot police, calming the excessive inflammation (the collateral damage) without completely disarming the defenders needed to clear the actual virus. And knowing how HMPV plays its tricks, how it jams the signals of our own "intelligence agents" (DCs), is vital for designing vaccines that can outsmart the virus, training our immune system to mount a response that's both powerful and precise, avoiding the devastating friendly fire. The most severe battles, often seen in those with weaker defenses to begin with, teach us the hardest lessons about what happens when this intricate, fiery dance goes terribly wrong.

When the Walls Are Breached: Calling in the Specialists

Imagine Human Metapneumovirus (HMPV) as an unwelcome intruder sneaking past our body's first line of security. It doesn't just trigger a general alarm; it prompts a call to the elite specialists – our adaptive immune system. This isn't just a brute force response; it's a highly coordinated operation with two main divisions: the ground troops (cell-mediated immunity led by T cells) and the intelligence and precision strike unit (humoral immunity, driven by B cells that become antibody factories) [Ref 1].

Think of T cells as having different roles on the battlefield. Cytotoxic T cells are the demolition experts, identifying cells hijacked by the virus and eliminating them to stop the enemy from multiplying. Helper T cells are the field commanders, directing the entire operation, motivating other defenders like B cells and cleanup crews (macrophages). Meanwhile, B cells, once activated, are like skilled artisans, crafting highly specific weapons – antibodies – designed precisely for HMPV [Ref 1]. These antibodies act like smart tags or targeted neutralizers; they can physically block the virus from entering our cells or mark infected cells for destruction, essentially painting a target on the enemy's back. Researchers have even identified the virus's specific "uniform" patches – proteins like F and G – that these antibody missiles lock onto, showcasing the system's incredible precision [e.g., Research by Skiadopoulos et al.].

The Protector Turns Aggressor: When Defense Causes Damage

But here's the twist: sometimes, this powerful defense force, in its zeal to eliminate the invader, causes significant "friendly fire." This phenomenon, known as immunopathology, is the dark side of our sophisticated immune response [Ref 6]. Instead of just clearing the virus and restoring peace, an over-enthusiastic or poorly controlled immune reaction can scorch the very territory it's meant to protect – our delicate lung tissue. This internal conflict can turn illnesses like bronchiolitis and pneumonia from manageable skirmishes into devastating battles, challenging the simple notion that immunity is purely beneficial.

Evidence paints a compelling picture: this self-inflicted damage is a major player in severe HMPV cases [Ref 6]. Why does this happen? One theory is a sluggish eviction process [Ref 6]. If the adaptive immune system can't swiftly kick HMPV out, the virus lingers, constantly poking the immune system. Imagine repeatedly sounding an alarm; eventually, the responders might become hyper-alert, overreacting and causing chaos. This sustained immune activation can lead to chronic inflammation, a pile-up of immune cells in the lungs that inadvertently damages the airways – like an army continuing to shell a town after the main threat has passed, hitting vital infrastructure.

Lessons from the Lab and the Bedside

Scientists use animal models – often mice and cotton rats – as simulators to understand these complex battle dynamics [Ref 6]. These studies have revealed that certain T cell squads, intended to be protective, can actually spearhead the attack on lung tissue during HMPV infection [Ref 6, e.g., studies by Graziani et al.]. Some experiments dramatically showed that removing specific T cell types could lessen lung damage and sickness in infected mice, even if the amount of virus didn't change much – directly pointing the finger at these cells for causing harm [General findings from HMPV mouse models]. It's also about communication breakdown; if the chemical signals (cytokines) guiding the immune response are unbalanced, leaning too heavily towards aggression, it can fuel tissue destruction instead of promoting efficient cleanup and repair.

Doctors see echoes of this in hospitals. A striking observation in children severely ill with HMPV is often lymphopenia – a noticeable drop in the number of circulating immune soldiers (T and B cells) in their blood [Ref 6]. It's like seeing troops disappear from the capital's streets. Why? They might be rushing en masse to the front lines (the inflamed lungs), they could be burning out and dying off after intense activation, or it might be a sign the infection itself is temporarily suppressing the entire defense system [Ref 6]. This drop in lymphocyte count is frequently noted in severe HMPV cases, sometimes correlating with the need for intensive care, suggesting it's a marker of the body struggling with this internal conflict [e.g., Clinical studies like those by Williams et al. or Cebey-López et al.].

Turning Understanding into Action

Knowing about this double-edged sword isn't just academic; it has real-world consequences:

Smarter Vaccines: This knowledge is crucial for designing HMPV vaccines that are safe and effective [Ref 6]. We learned harsh lessons from RSV (HMPV's close relative), where early vaccine attempts tragically primed the immune system incorrectly, making the illness worse upon actual infection. The goal for HMPV vaccines is to train the immune system to be a disciplined, effective force, not an unregulated militia prone to causing collateral damage [Ref 6].

Identifying the Vulnerable: Realizing that severity depends on both the virus and the host's reaction helps us think about who might be most at risk. Perhaps subtle differences in our genetic makeup or underlying health conditions make some individuals' immune systems more likely to overreact. While not yet a standard tool, tracking things like lymphocyte counts might one day help doctors gauge a patient's risk of heading towards severe, immune-driven disease.

Future Treatment Ideas: Currently, we mostly offer supportive care for HMPV. But understanding the immunopathology opens doors for potential future treatments. In critical situations where inflammation seems to be driving the illness, perhaps highly targeted therapies could gently dial back the excessive immune response (think specific cytokine blockers or carefully judged corticosteroids). This is a delicate balancing act – you don't want to disable the defenses needed to fight the virus – and requires much more research, but it's a potential avenue born from understanding this immune paradox [Conceptual application]. Imagine a critically ill child; recognizing the signs of potential immunopathology might subtly shift how doctors manage their supportive care, aiming to minimize anything that could further provoke the inflammatory storm.

In the end, our adaptive immune response to HMPV is a gripping story of defense and potential self-sabotage. T cells and B cells are essential heroes in this fight, but under certain conditions, they can contribute to the very lung damage they are supposed to prevent [Ref 1, Ref 6]. Untangling this complex relationship, through ongoing scientific detective work and careful clinical observation, is key to protecting patients better and designing truly safe interventions like vaccines.

Okay, let's breathe some life into this intricate process. Imagine your airways not just as tubes, but as delicate, vital corridors lined with a living tapestry – the epithelial cells. This is where our story begins, not with a sterile "viral particle," but with an unseen trespasser, maybe an RSV or Flu virus, landing softly on this precious lining (Ref 1).

This isn't just a landing; it's an invasion. The virus, a microscopic hijacker, forces its way into these guardian cells. It doesn't ask permission; it rewires the cell's own machinery to churn out copies of itself. Think of it like a rogue agent taking over a crucial control room. The cell, overwhelmed and damaged, might simply die, break apart (necrosis), or initiate a self-destruct sequence (apoptosis), shedding itself like a crumbling brick from a wall, leaving gaps in the protective barrier (Ref 1, 6). Scientists have even peeked through powerful microscopes to witness this aftermath – airways stripped bare after a viral siege (Evidence: Aherne et al.).

This cellular breakdown isn't silent. It screams for help. The injured cells and the presence of the viral intruders send out desperate signals – chemical flares like IL-6, IL-8, and TNF-alpha (Ref 17). These signals rally the body's emergency response team: a flood of immune cells (neutrophils, lymphocytes, macrophages) rushes to the scene (Ref 1, 17). Imagine firefighters and paramedics converging, sirens blazing. Tests on fluid washed from deep within the lungs of sick patients confirm this rush – levels of these alarm signals, especially the neutrophil-attracting IL-8, can skyrocket, acting as a measure of how fierce the battle is (Fact: IL-8 levels can surge hundreds of times higher).

But here's the tragic irony: this valiant defense force, while fighting the virus, creates chaos of its own. The sheer number of responder cells causes the airway walls – the corridors themselves – to swell and thicken, like crowds jamming a hallway during an emergency (Ref 6, 17). This inflammation physically squishes the open space, making the passageway narrower.

At the same time, the alarm signals push the airway's mucus factories (goblet cells and glands) into frantic overdrive (Ref 6). It's not just more mucus; it's often a thicker, stickier goo designed to trap invaders but ends up creating biological traffic jams in the already constricted tunnels. To make matters worse, the ongoing inflammation can make the airway muscles twitchy and prone to sudden constriction (bronchial hyper-responsiveness or BHR), like a sensitive alarm system triggered by the slightest disturbance, clamping down the airway even further (Ref 17). Specific inflammatory molecules released during the fight, like leukotrienes, are known culprits behind this twitchiness.

So, what's the result of this internal drama? You have crumbling cell debris, swollen and inflamed airway walls, excessive sticky mucus, and potentially hyper-sensitive, constricting muscles. It's a perfect storm brewing inside these tiny tubes, leading to a critical blockage (Ref 6, 17). This is especially dangerous for infants and toddlers, whose airways are already pencil-thin – imagine a 4-5mm wide passage suddenly reduced by swelling and mucus! (Fact: Infant airways are tiny, making blockage much easier).

This internal gridlock is what you feel and hear as sickness (Ref 6, 17):

The Cough: Your body's forceful attempt to clear the debris, the sticky mucus, and soothe the irritation.

The Wheeze: That high-pitched whistle? It's the sound of air desperately squeezing through the severely narrowed, obstructed passageways.
Rapid Breathing (Tachypnea) & Shortness of Breath (Dyspnea): Your body working overtime, gasping faster and harder, trying to pull in enough oxygen past the blockages. It's a physical struggle against resistance.
Low Blood Oxygen (Hypoxia): When the blockage gets too severe, oxygen simply can't get through the jammed corridors and inflamed air sacs (alveoli) to reach the bloodstream where it's needed. The vital exchange is impaired.

Doctors can often "see" echoes of this internal battle on X-rays or CT scans (Ref 7). The swollen airway walls might appear as ghostly rings ("peribronchial cuffing"). Areas where the lung tissue itself is caught in the crossfire – filled with inflammatory fluid, mucus plugs, or collapsed air sacs – show up as shadowy patches or infiltrates (Ref 7).

Bringing it Home: A Tiny Fighter's Story

Picture an 8-month-old baby rushed into the ER. He's breathing fast, you can hear a distinct wheeze, and the skin around his ribs sucks in with every desperate gasp (retractions). A quick test confirms RSV is the culprit (bronchiolitis). Here's the microscopic drama playing out inside him:

Invasion: RSV stormed his tiny airway lining, causing cells to break down.

The Siege: His immune system responded fiercely, but this led to significant swelling in his already small bronchioles.

The Goo: Mucus production went haywire, adding thick plugs to the swelling.

The Blockade: Swollen walls + mucus + debris = critically narrowed airways (maybe squeezed from 4mm down to just 1-2mm!).

The Struggle: The wheeze is air fighting through those tiny gaps. The rapid breathing and retractions show his immense effort. Sadly, the blockage is so bad, he's struggling to get enough oxygen (hypoxia).

The Evidence: An X-ray likely shows hyperinflated lungs (air trapped behind blockages), thickened airway walls, and maybe fuzzy patches of inflammation, confirming the chaos within.

Understanding this journey – from a single virus breaching the gates to the body's overwhelming response causing the very symptoms of illness – isn't just academic. It's the key to helping that baby breathe easier, guiding doctors to use oxygen, clear the mucus, and support the tiny patient through the internal storm. It's a profound reminder of the delicate balance within our own bodies.

The Clinical Face of HMPV: Spectrum of Manifestations from Mild Cold to Critical Illness

Meet HMPV: The Respiratory Shapeshifter

Imagine a microscopic entity, relatively new to our scientific acquaintance (only stepping into the spotlight in 2001!), yet already proving itself a master of disguise in the world of respiratory illnesses. This isn't your average, predictable bug. Human Metapneumovirus, or HMPV, doesn't just cause one kind of sick; it has a whole repertoire, a stunningly wide spectrum of effects that can touch anyone, from the perfectly healthy to the critically ill. Think of it less like a simple cold virus and more like a character actor, capable of playing vastly different roles depending on the stage (our bodies) and the audience (our immune systems).

The Silent Role: HMPV the Ghost

Sometimes, HMPV is the ultimate wallflower. It can slip into our airways – nose, throat, lungs – and just... hang out. Sensitive tests can pick up its genetic fingerprint in people who feel completely fine, showing zero signs of illness. Like finding footprints on a path long after someone has passed, detecting HMPV doesn't automatically mean you're sick or even contagious. It can be a silent passenger, a ghost in our respiratory machine, its presence noted but not felt. Why it sometimes chooses this stealth mode is still a bit of a mystery researchers are untangling, but it reminds us that the relationship between viruses and humans is complex – not always a battle, sometimes just co-existence.

The Annoying Cameo: HMPV as the Common Cold Impersonator

More often, HMPV auditions for the role we all know too well: the common cold. It can bring on that familiar, unwelcome troupe of symptoms – the nagging cough, the low-grade fever that makes you feel 'off,' the endlessly runny nose, maybe a scratchy throat. If you caught an HMPV cold, you'd likely blame it on any number of usual suspects. It blends right in. However, while it definitely contributes to the global burden of sniffles, it's not the headliner. That title usually belongs to the Rhinovirus family, the undisputed superstars of the common cold world. HMPV is more like a recurring guest star, responsible for a smaller, but still significant, slice of those "under the weather" days (think maybe 1 in 10 or 1 in 20 colds, compared to Rhinovirus's starring role in potentially half of them).

The Dramatic Lead: HMPV the Lung Invader

But HMPV has a much more serious, dramatic side, and this is where it truly commands attention, often with devastating consequences. When it decides to go beyond a simple head cold and delve deeper into the lungs, it becomes a major player in serious Lower Respiratory Tract Infections. This is where it earns its reputation, primarily by causing:

Bronchiolitis: Inflaming the tiny, delicate airways deep within the lungs, making breathing difficult, especially for the smallest among us.

Pneumonia: Infecting the lung tissue itself, a serious condition requiring significant medical care.

This dangerous transformation is most likely to happen in those whose defenses are not at their peak:

Tiny Infants: Their brand-new immune systems are still learning the ropes.

Older Adults: Whose immune responses may have slowed down over time.

People with Compromised Immunity: Individuals battling other conditions or undergoing treatments (like transplants) that weaken their body's guards.

In hospitals worldwide, HMPV consistently shows up as a leading cause of lung infections that put kids in beds, second often only to the infamous RSV (Respiratory Syncytial Virus). Studies show it's behind a significant chunk (maybe 5% to 15%) of these serious pediatric cases. It can sweep through nursing homes causing severe pneumonia, and for transplant patients, an HMPV infection can be a prolonged, dangerous ordeal.

Why Understanding HMPV's Many Faces Matters:

Knowing this virus's chameleon-like nature isn't just academic; it has real-world impact:

In the ER: When a baby arrives struggling to breathe, doctors know that while RSV is common, HMPV is a very real possibility. Pinpointing HMPV helps guide treatment and manage expectations (sometimes HMPV hospital stays are even longer). It also helps keep vulnerable patients safe by preventing spread within the hospital.

Protecting Public Health: Health agencies track HMPV like weather forecasters track storms. They watch its seasonal patterns (usually late winter/spring) to help hospitals anticipate surges, especially in pediatric intensive care units, ensuring resources are ready.

The Quest for a Shield: Because HMPV can hit the young and vulnerable so hard, and we lack specific knockout medicines for it, it's a prime target for vaccine developers.

The goal? To create a shield, particularly for infants and the elderly, protecting them from HMPV's potentially life-threatening roles.

In Essence:

HMPV is far more than just another virus. It's a respiratory entity with a complex personality – capable of being an unseen presence, a minor nuisance, or a formidable threat. Recognizing its full range, from silent guest to dangerous invader, is crucial for doctors treating patients, scientists developing defenses, and all of us navigating the world of respiratory health. It's a reminder that even the smallest things can have a vast and varied impact on human lives.

Decoding Your Body's S.O.S.: Recognizing the Familiar Tune of Respiratory Bugs

Think of it like this: when those seasonal bugs decide to pay a visit, our bodies start sending out distress signals. Understanding the typical "song" they sing can help us figure out what's going on, whether it's time to call the doctor, or just time for tea and sympathy. While everyone's experience is their own personal remix, there's definitely a common beat, though the rhythm section might sound different in a kid versus a grown-up.

The Headliner: That Persistent Cough

Leading the charge, almost always, is the cough. It's not just a minor throat-clearing; this is often the main event, the symptom that sticks around like an over-enthusiastic party guest. Imagine the soundtrack of winter – that rhythmic coughing is hard to miss! Research backs this up, showing it steals the spotlight in a whopping 80% to 90% of cases when these bugs hit. It's the body's forceful attempt to clear the decks, and boy, does it make its presence known.

The Annoying Sidekick: The Stuffy, Runny Nose

Close on the cough's heels comes that feeling of being utterly stuffed up, or the alternative – a nose that runs like a leaky faucet (doctors call it rhinorrhea, we call it annoying). This nasal nuisance shows up in over 70% of people feeling unwell, playing a big part in that general "ugh, I'm sick" sensation. It's the body trying to flush things out, but it mostly feels like a traffic jam in your sinuses.

Fever: The Age-Sensitive Alarm Bell

Now, fever is where things get really interesting, acting like a different kind of alarm depending on your age. Think of a little kid's immune system as being new on the job – it often reacts LOUDLY. Fevers are super common in children, maybe popping up in half to even 80% of sick little ones. But in adults? Their immune systems are more seasoned veterans; they've seen things. So, a fever might only show up less than 4% of the time. This is crucial! Public health folks often watch for "fever plus cough" (calling it "influenza-like illness") to track bugs like the flu. But if you're an adult feeling rough without a temperature, don't assume you're in the clear – your body might just be fighting the battle more quietly.

The Supporting Cast: When Other Symptoms Join the Party

Beyond the big three, a whole crew of other symptoms can show up, making the picture more complex.

Wheezing or feeling short of breath? That's a sign the trouble might be heading deeper into the lungs –

definitely something to watch, especially in babies or people with asthma.

Sore throat? Yep, very common, like sandpaper decided to take up residence.

Lost your voice (laryngitis)? Or hear that seal-bark cough from a child (croup)? That suggests the inflammation is hitting the voice box.

Pink eye (conjunctivitis) or an earache (otitis media)? Sometimes the infection likes to spread to the neighbours.

Headache and that overall feeling of being completely drained (malaise)? These are the systemic reminders that your whole body is busy fighting.

Even tummy troubles or a rash can occasionally appear, though they're usually less common characters in this particular play.

Different Ages, Different Scripts

Remember that age difference with fever? It applies elsewhere too. While kids often present with that dramatic cough and fever combo, studies suggest adults might complain more about the stuffy nose, sore throat, sheer exhaustion, and those lovely muscle aches that make you feel ancient. It's like the illness follows a slightly different script depending on the actor's age.

Why Knowing the Script Matters: Real-World Scenes

Understanding these patterns isn't just trivia; it's incredibly practical:

The Doctor's Office Detective Work: A pediatrician hears a high fever, hacking cough, and wheezing in a toddler. Their mind might jump to certain viruses common in kids (like RSV). Compare that to an adult calling in, mainly complaining of feeling wiped out, headachy, with a sore, stuffy throat but no fever. The doctor uses these different "symptom stories" to guide their thinking and decide on next steps, perhaps ordering different tests based on the clues.

Keeping Tabs on Community Health: Those public health officials tracking "fever + cough"? They're using this symptom knowledge as an early warning system, helping communities prepare and respond when illnesses start spreading like wildfire.

The Telemedicine Challenge: When you're talking to a doctor through a screen, they rely heavily on your description. Knowing the typical symptom set, and how it varies, helps them piece together the puzzle and give you the best advice, even from miles away.

So, while a cough and sniffles might seem simple, they're part of a complex set of signals. Learning to read them – including the variations and the age-related nuances uncovered by careful research – helps everyone, from doctors making diagnoses to public health teams keeping us safe, and even helps you understand what your body might be trying to tell you during that unwelcome seasonal visit.

When a Common Cold Becomes a Thief of Breath: Understanding RSV's Critical Turn

We've all known the sniffles, the cough, the tired drag of a common cold. Most of the time, Respiratory Syncytial Virus (RSV) is just that – an unwelcome visitor that soon departs. But for some, this seemingly ordinary virus transforms into something far more menacing. Imagine that familiar cough deepening, the breath catching, turning into a desperate fight for air. For the tiniest infants, the frail elderly, or those already battling chronic illness, RSV can unleash a terrifying assault on the lungs, demanding the highest levels of medical intervention [1, 2]. This isn't just about feeling unwell; it's about a sudden plunge into a respiratory crisis, a stark reminder of RSV's hidden power and the immense pressure it puts on our intensive care lifelines [3].

The Tiny Lungs' Struggle: Infant Bronchiolitis

Picture the most delicate airways imaginable – the whisper-thin passages deep inside a baby's lungs, barely wider than a thread. Now, imagine those passages inflamed, swollen shut, choked with sticky mucus [1, 5]. This is RSV bronchiolitis, the virus's most feared attack on infants, especially those under six months or born too soon [4]. Breathing becomes an agonizing effort. You see it in the frantic rise and fall of their tiny chests, the skin pulling tight around their ribs with each gasp (retractions), hear it in the strained wheeze, and know it by the frightening dip in their oxygen levels [6]. It's a desperate physiological cry for help. A heartbreaking number of these little ones hospitalized with RSV need more than just oxygen; they need advanced breathing support in the Pediatric Intensive Care Unit (PICU) [7, 8]. While numbers fluctuate, seeing 2-3% or even more of hospitalized babies needing intensive care specifically for RSV paints a stark picture of its potential severity [22, 9].

When Lungs Become a Battleground: Adult Pneumonia and ARDS

For adults, particularly older individuals or those whose bodies are already taxed by chronic heart or lung disease (like COPD or asthma) or weakened defenses, severe RSV often lands its blow as aggressive pneumonia [10]. The virus doesn't just irritate; it injures the lung tissue itself, inflaming the delicate air sacs where life-giving oxygen exchange happens [5, 11]. In the most critical scenarios, the lungs seem to wage war on themselves, leading to Acute Respiratory Distress Syndrome (ARDS) [1, 5]. This isn't just pneumonia; it's a catastrophic lung failure. Widespread inflammation causes fluid to swamp the air sacs, making it nearly impossible for the lungs to do their job [12]. Think of a sponge utterly waterlogged – that's ARDS. RSV is increasingly unmasked as a major culprit behind severe, community-acquired pneumonia hospitalizations in adults [13]. And when adults are hospitalized with RSV, the need for intensive care spikes dramatically – sometimes 10-20% or even higher, especially if they have underlying health issues, landing in the ICU far more often than children [14, 22]. Some studies focusing solely on the sickest adults show roughly 1 in 8 hospitalized RSV patients needing ICU care [22].

The ICU Lifeline: Fighting for Every Breath

When breathing fails, whether from choked infant airways or overwhelmed adult lungs, the Intensive Care Unit becomes the critical command center [5]. The mission is clear: support the body's need for oxygen, buy precious time for the lungs to heal [15]. It often starts simply, with extra oxygen [7]. But frequently, the battle escalates. High-flow nasal cannula (HFNC) therapy arrives, bathing the airways in warm, humidified, oxygen-rich air, a powerful helping hand that can sometimes stave off more invasive measures [16]. Yet, when the patient is simply too exhausted to breathe, or oxygen levels remain perilously low despite HFNC, the ultimate support becomes necessary: mechanical ventilation [5, 17]. A breathing tube is gently placed, and a machine takes over the vital, rhythmic work of breathing, a vital alliance between technology and the human body [17]. In ICUs grappling with severe RSV, this isn't rare. Studies show a significant portion, sometimes over half of ICU RSV patients (especially adults with ARDS), rely on these machines [18, 19]. And for the absolute direst cases of ARDS, where even ventilators struggle, the extraordinary measure of ECMO –

oxygenating the blood outside the body – might be the final safety net, a complex feat reserved for specialized centers [20].

Faces Behind the Fight: Stories from the Brink

The Smallest Warrior: Imagine a two-month-old baby, born a little early, whose small cough, picked up from a sibling, rapidly worsens. In the ER, their tiny chest heaves, oxygen levels plummet (85%), and the diagnosis is severe RSV bronchiolitis [6, 8]. Even high-flow oxygen isn't enough; the baby tires, breaths become shallow, carbon dioxide climbs – a sign the body can no longer keep up [17]. The next step is the PICU, a breathing tube, and the steady rhythm of the ventilator, breathing for them until the inflammation calms [7, 17]. This isn't just a statistic; it's a family's world turned upside down, mirroring countless documented battles in pediatric critical care [9].

The Elder's Ordeal: Picture a 70-year-old man, managing his COPD, caught in a community RSV wave [10, 13]. His familiar cough deepens, breathlessness intensifies, and within 48 hours, he's in severe respiratory distress. Chest X-rays show lungs clouded by pneumonia rapidly progressing to ARDS [1, 12]. He's rushed to the ICU, immediately needing intubation and the powerful support of a ventilator working against stiff, injured lungs [18]. His recovery is slow, marked by setbacks in weaning from the machine – a difficult journey reflecting the harsh reality of RSV-induced ARDS in older adults, often documented in critical care reports [14, 19].

The Echo of RSV's Severity

RSV may wear the mask of a common cold, but beneath it lies the potential for profound, life-threatening respiratory failure – be it the suffocating grip of bronchiolitis in infants or the devastating lung injury of pneumonia and ARDS in adults [1, 5]. The stark rates of ICU admission, especially among adults, and the frequent, urgent need for mechanical ventilation underscore the critical edge of this virus [17, 22]. Each severe case is not just a medical challenge; it's a human story of vulnerability, a testament to the strain on critical care resources, and a powerful call for continued vigilance, better prevention, and the unwavering pursuit of rapid recognition and care [3, 21].

When the Ground Beneath You Shifts: Worsening Chronic Conditions

For someone living with the constant vigilance of asthma or COPD, breathing is already a careful negotiation. Their airways are sensitive territories. Introduce a common cold or flu virus, and it's like throwing a lit match into dry tinder (Ref 6). That carefully managed stability? It can vanish. Suddenly, the familiar wheeze tightens into a desperate fight for air, a flare-up – or "exacerbation" in doctor-speak – that feels like a betrayal by their own body. Research whispers (loudly, in fact) that these viruses are the villains behind a huge chunk of these sudden downturns (Evidence: Johnston SL et al., NEJM 1995; Wedzicha JA et al., Thorax 2000). It's not just discomfort; it's a scramble for rescue inhalers, urgent calls to the doctor, maybe even the jarring lights and sterile scent of an emergency room. It's the frustrating reality of a simple sniffle hijacking their life.

The Tiny Blockade: Echoes in the Ear

Think about the head's plumbing – specifically, that tiny canal, the Eustachian tube, linking the back of your throat to the middle ear. It's usually an unnoticed pathway for air and drainage. But when a respiratory virus stirs up inflammation and mucus like a chaotic construction crew

(Ref 11), this tube can get blocked. Suddenly, the middle ear becomes a stuffy, sealed-off room, perfect for moisture to gather and unwelcome guests – bacteria or the virus itself – to throw a party. This is the story behind countless childhood earaches (otitis media) that often follow a cold (Evidence: Heikkinen T et al., NEJM 1999). Picture a little one, finally getting over sniffles and coughs, suddenly spiking a fever, tugging at their ear, inconsolable – the echo of the respiratory bug creating a new pocket of misery.

An Open Door for Unwanted Guests: Secondary Infections

Sometimes, the initial viral attack does more than just make you feel lousy; it weakens the castle walls. The virus can rough up the delicate lining of the lungs, paralyze the tiny hairs (cilia) meant to sweep away debris, and generally distract the local security forces (immune cells). This disruption creates an opportunistic opening (Ref 22). Bacteria that might normally be kept in check, like Streptococcus pneumoniae, see their chance and launch a secondary invasion, leading to bacterial pneumonia. It's a cruel twist: just as someone starts feeling they've turned a corner from the flu, they're hit again, harder, with high fevers, a chest rattling with coughs, and the shadow of pneumonia on an X-ray. History, especially during devastating flu pandemics, reminds us how deadly this one-two punch can be (Evidence: Morens DM et al., J Infect Dis 2008).

The Body's Defenses in Disarray: Shifts in Blood

Deep within, the battle affects the troops. During some viral respiratory campaigns, the numbers of key immune soldiers called lymphocytes can drop significantly – a state called lymphopenia (Ref 6). Think of it as the body's special forces being depleted or exhausted. This isn't just a footnote in a blood test; observations, especially during the intense fight against COVID-19, showed that a deeper plunge in lymphocyte counts often signaled a tougher battle ahead, hinting at a more severe illness (Evidence: Huang C et al., Lancet 2020). It's a quiet signal from the blood, reflecting the scale of the internal struggle.

Rare Tremors in the Control Center and Engine Room: Neurological & Cardiac Events

While uncommon, the ripples can sometimes reach the most sensitive areas: the nervous system and the heart. In rare instances, a respiratory virus might be linked to bewildering neurological events – seizures striking without a fever, a sudden loss of balance and coordination (ataxia), or even inflammation clouding the brain itself (encephalitis) (Ref 6, Evidence: Ekstrand JJ et al., Clin Infect Dis 2010). Imagine the fear when, recovering from the flu, someone experiences sudden confusion or a child develops unexplained seizures. Similarly, though thankfully very rare, the heart muscle can become inflamed (myocarditis) in the aftermath of certain infections (Ref 29, Evidence: Ukimura A et al., Circ J 2012) – a serious whisper of the virus's potential reach.

The Mystery: Direct Hit or Friendly Fire?

This leads to a fascinating and critical question: How does a lung virus cause trouble in the brain or heart (Ref 6; Insight 6.3.1)? Is the virus itself a master infiltrator, directly invading these distant tissues? Or is it more complex – is the body's own immune response, triggered by the virus but becoming overzealous, inadvertently causing damage elsewhere? Growing evidence leans towards this "friendly fire" hypothesis in many cases. The inflammation intended to fight the virus might spill over, harming unintended targets. Knowing the difference is crucial. A direct viral attack might need antivirals, while immune-mediated damage might call for therapies to calm the immune system (Ref 6). It's like determining if the damage is from the enemy's bomb or from the chaotic aftermath of your own defenses.

In essence, a respiratory illness can be far more than a cough and sniffle. It's a potential catalyst, capable of triggering flare-ups in vulnerable airways, opening doors for bacterial follow-ons, subtly shifting our internal defenses, and, rarely, causing unexpected crises in distant parts of our bodily ecosystem, possibly through the very fire of our own immune response. Recognizing this intricate web of possibilities is key to truly understanding – and caring for – the whole person behind the cough.

Identifying the Culprit: HMPV Diagnostic Strategies and Interpretation in 2025

Cracking the Code: When Coughs Confuse, Molecules Give Clarity

It starts with a familiar sound: a cough. Then maybe a fever, the struggle for a full breath. Especially when the seasons turn, a wave of respiratory misery can wash over homes, schools, and workplaces. Is it the flu? A common cold? RSV? Or could it be the lesser-known but still potent Human Metapneumovirus (HMPV)? To the worried parent, the overwhelmed doctor, or the person feeling rotten, the symptoms often blur into one confusing picture. Trying to guess the culprit based on symptoms alone is like trying to identify a bird solely by its distant song – tricky, and often wrong.

This is where science steps out of the lab and offers a powerful flashlight in the fog: molecular detection. Forget guesswork; we're talking about reading the virus's own signature. The undisputed champion in the HMPV identification ring is RT-PCR (Reverse Transcription Polymerase Chain Reaction). Think of it as the master detective for HMPV. It doesn't just look at symptoms; it hunts for the virus's unique genetic fingerprint – its RNA.

Imagine the process: First, we gently coax the virus's delicate RNA instructions into a sturdier DNA format. Then, the real magic happens. PCR acts like a super-powered photocopier, but only for the HMPV genetic code. It finds tiny fragments of the virus in a sample (like from a simple nose swab) and makes millions, even billions, of copies. Suddenly, even the faintest whisper of HMPV becomes a roar that machines can easily detect. It's incredibly sensitive, catching infections that older methods like trying to grow the virus in a dish (culture) or basic antigen tests might miss entirely. RT-PCR delivers a clear, confident "Yes, HMPV is here" or "No, look elsewhere."

But modern medicine rarely deals with just one suspect. What if it isn't HMPV? Testing for HMPV, then RSV, then flu, then COVID-19... playing that kind of diagnostic whack-a-mole is agonizingly slow and eats up precious time and resources. Enter the Multiplex Marvels – the sophisticated diagnostic panels.

Picture this: Instead of one detective focusing on one suspect, you have a whole team simultaneously interrogating all the usual suspects from a single clue (the patient sample). That's a multiplex PCR panel. It takes the pinpoint accuracy of RT-PCR and applies it across the board. In one test, it can search for HMPV plus RSV, Influenza A and B, various parainfluenza troublemakers, adenoviruses, rhinoviruses (the common cold culprits), seasonal coronaviruses, and the pandemic headliner, SARS-CoV-2. It's like trading a single key for a master key that unlocks the identity of nearly any common respiratory virus.

The payoff? It's huge, touching everything from the bedside to broad public health:

Cutting Through the Symptom Chaos: No more agonizing delays while testing one virus after another. Multiplex panels deliver a panoramic view of the potential culprits quickly. This swift clarity is pure gold, especially when dealing with fragile patients like babies, seniors, or those with weakened immune systems. Knowing the enemy fast means you can fight back smarter, sooner.

Treatment Tailored, Not Guessed: Information is power. Confirming Influenza means potent antiviral drugs like oseltamivir can be deployed early, when they work best.

Identifying HMPV or RSV, for which we lack specific everyday antivirals, means focusing on what truly helps – fluids, oxygen support if needed – and crucially, avoiding treatments that won't work.

Smarter Defense Against Spread: In hospitals or care homes, knowing exactly what's circulating is critical. Is it HMPV, flu, or COVID-19? The answer dictates the battle plan: specific isolation tactics, the right protective gear, and how to group patients (cohorting) to prevent turning a ward into a viral mixing bowl. Multiplex results are the intel needed for targeted infection control.

Guardians of Our Antibiotics: This might be the unsung superpower. Viruses don't respond to antibiotics. Period. Yet, desperate for answers and solutions, antibiotics are often mistakenly prescribed for viral illnesses. Multiplex panels, by firmly pointing the finger at a virus like HMPV, give doctors the confidence to say "No" to unnecessary antibiotics. In a world grappling with the terrifying rise of antibiotic resistance – a crisis fueled by overuse – these tests are vital shields, preserving the power of medicines we desperately need.

And there's even another layer: some advanced RT-PCR tests (qRT-PCR) can not only detect the virus but estimate how much of it is present (the viral load). While this "volume knob" isn't typically used to guide day-to-day HMPV treatment, it's invaluable for researchers tracking how the virus behaves, understanding if higher loads mean worse illness, or monitoring how well experimental treatments are working.

See it in Action:

The Wheezing Baby: A tiny infant struggles to breathe in the ER. Is it RSV? Something else? The multiplex panel quickly comes back: HMPV positive, everything else negative. Diagnosis clear. Treatment focuses on support (oxygen, maybe fluids). Parents are reassured antibiotics aren't needed. Everyone breathes a little easier (metaphorically, at least).

The Nursing Home Outbreak: Coughs echo down the halls. Fear of flu or COVID looms. Multiplex testing reveals HMPV is the uninvited guest. Immediately, staff implement the right precautions for HMPV, cohort affected residents, and communicate clearly, preventing widespread panic and unnecessary lockdowns.

Flu Season Strategy: An older patient with heart issues develops severe symptoms. Time is critical. The panel flags Influenza A, ruling out HMPV, RSV, and COVID. Antiviral medication starts immediately, potentially warding off severe complications for this vulnerable individual.

In essence, molecular detection, powered by the precision of RT-PCR and the efficiency of multiplex panels, has dragged respiratory diagnostics out of the era of educated guesses and into an age of molecular certainty. It gives doctors rapid, reliable answers, leading to better care, wiser resource use, and a crucial defense against the looming threat of antibiotic resistance. It's about shining a bright, revealing light on the invisible microbial world, one accurate diagnosis at a time.

Beyond the PCR Hype: Meet the Diagnostic World's Unsung Heroes (and Understand Their Limits)

We hear a lot about PCR tests – the super-sensitive sleuths of the diagnostic world, amazing at sniffing out the faintest genetic trail of a virus. They're fantastic, no doubt. But thinking PCR is the only player is like saying a detective only needs high-tech surveillance and forgets about quick street checks or deep forensic analysis. Sometimes, you need a different kind of expert, and that's where antigen tests and viral cultures step into the spotlight, each with its own unique talent and, yes, its own quirks.

Antigen Tests: The Need-for-Speed Crew

Imagine this: it's peak flu season, your clinic is buzzing, and someone walks in feeling rough. You need answers, fast. Enter the rapid antigen test, the diagnostic equivalent of a quick field report. In just 15-30 minutes (Ref 26), you get a yes/no signal. That speed is pure gold. It means doctors can decide right now if antivirals (which work best early) are needed or if someone needs to head home and isolate, stopping potential spread in its tracks (Ref 26). Think pharmacies, workplaces, even your own home – antigen tests bring answers to where life happens. They're the point-of-care champions, designed for immediate action.

But here's the trade-off, the catch: speed often means sacrificing depth. Antigen tests look for specific protein chunks on the virus's surface. To get a positive, you need a decent amount of virus hanging around (Ref 26). If the virus is just starting its invasion, or if someone doesn't have many symptoms (and maybe less virus), the antigen test might just miss it. It's like trying to spot someone in a dimly lit room with a quick flashlight beam – you might easily miss them if they're lurking in the shadows. This means a negative antigen test isn't always a definitive "all clear," especially if you suspect an early infection (Ref 26). It's a great first look, but maybe not the final word for ruling something out.

Viral Culture: The Old-School Sage with Deep Insights

Now, let's shift gears to viral culture. This isn't your everyday test; it's more like the meticulous, old-school researcher, the one who doesn't just find clues but actually brings the culprit (the live, replicating virus) back to the lab for intense study (Ref 1, 3, 26, 38). Why bother with this slow, complex process? Because sometimes, you need to know more than just "is the virus present?". You need to know if it's alive and kicking.

This is absolutely critical for the big picture stuff. When a new flu strain pops up, how do scientists figure out how dangerous it is, if our drugs will work against it (Ref 1, 3), or how to update the vaccine (Ref 38)? They culture the virus – grow it, isolate it, and study its behaviour. Researchers testing new antiviral drugs need culture to see if their compound actually stops the virus in its tracks (Ref 1, 3). Viral culture is the bedrock for understanding viruses, tracking their evolution, and preparing our defenses.

But for diagnosing sick patients quickly? Viral culture is mostly out of the running. It's slow – taking days, sometimes weeks, for results (Ref 26). Imagine waiting that long for answers when someone's seriously ill! Plus, it's demanding work, needing special labs with high safety measures (think hazmat suits for nasty bugs) and skilled scientists (Ref 1, 3). It can even be less sensitive than PCR sometimes, because you need viable, living virus in the sample, and it needs to survive the journey to the lab and grow happily in its new cell-line home (Ref 26). It's invaluable for research, but clinically impractical for rapid patient care (Ref 1, 3, 26, 38).

Choosing the Right Tool for the Job

So, while the speedy antigen test gives us crucial quick checks (just remember its potential blind spots), and the methodical viral culture provides irreplaceable depth for science and public health (though it's far too slow for routine diagnosis), PCR often remains the clinical workhorse (Ref 1, 3, 26, 38). Its blend of high sensitivity and reasonable speed makes it the go-to for reliably detecting viral footprints when accurate diagnosis is key for treating patients.

It's not about one test being universally "better" – it's about understanding what each tool does best and where its boundaries lie. Knowing this helps us use these powerful diagnostic allies wisely, whether we're managing a personal illness, a clinic caseload, or a global pandemic.

Serology: Listening to the Body's Echoes

Think of your immune system as a vigilant defender. When a microscopic intruder – a virus or bacterium – shows up, the defenders sound the alarm and eventually create specific "memory markers" called antibodies. Serology is the science dedicated to finding and understanding these markers, primarily swimming in our blood serum. It's less about catching the invader in the act, and more about finding the molecular footprints left behind.

Scientists use clever tools, like the workhorse technique ELISA, which acts like a highly specific scanner, searching for particular antibody signatures. Two key signatures they look for are IgM and IgG.

IgM: The Recent News Bulletin. Think of IgM as the first, urgent alert. It pops up relatively quickly after an infection starts – maybe days or weeks – shouting, "Hey, something new is happening right now, or just happened!" But like breaking news, its intensity fades over a few months.

IgG: The Historical Record. IgG is like the detailed entry logged in the history books. It arrives a bit later than IgM but sticks around much longer – years, sometimes even a lifetime. Finding IgG says, "This person met this germ before," signifying past exposure or the long-lasting protection offered by immunity, perhaps from a previous illness or a vaccine.

Unlocking History and Mapping the Present

Before we had lightning-fast genetic tests, serology was the ultimate detective for figuring out what swept through a community, long after the fevers cooled and coughs subsided. Scientists could pull out old, stored blood samples and, like biological archaeologists, map the spread of forgotten outbreaks, painting pictures of past epidemics.

This power to look back is precisely why serology is still a superstar in public health today. Its main gig? Seroprevalence studies. Imagine trying to understand how far a wildfire really spread, not just counting the houses that burned down. Serology does this for diseases. By testing blood from a cross-section of people, researchers can estimate how many individuals actually encountered a germ, including those who never felt sick or had only mild symptoms.

Remember the early days of COVID-19? Official case counts were just the tip of the iceberg. Serology studies pulled back the curtain, revealing that far more people had been infected than anyone realized based on diagnostic tests alone. One big US study suggested maybe 10 hidden infections for every confirmed case! This kind of intel is gold – it helps us grasp how diseases really move, who's most vulnerable, and the true scale of a health challenge.

Serology is also our go-to tool for gauging a community's immune shield. Are enough people protected against measles to keep it cornered? Are COVID-19 vaccines building a strong wall of defense across different age groups? By measuring IgG levels across a population, health officials can see if our collective armor – built through past infections or vaccination campaigns – is strong enough. If immunity seems to be dipping (like needing >90-95% protection for measles!), serology results can sound the call for booster shots or targeted vaccination efforts. We saw this happen in real-time with COVID-19 vaccines, where studies tracking antibody levels helped fine-tune dosing and booster strategies.

The Catch: Why Serology Isn't Great for the Doctor's Office Visit

For all its epidemiological brilliance, serology stumbles when it comes to diagnosing someone who is sick right now. Why? It's all about timing.

Our immune system needs time to build those detectable antibodies. There's a lag – the "window period" – between when you get infected and when tests like IgM or IgG turn positive. You could be actively sick and contagious, but a serology test done too early might come back negative, offering false reassurance. For many infections, you might need to wait 5-10 days after symptoms start for IgM to reliably show up, and even longer for IgG. That delay is a deal-breaker when a doctor needs answers now to decide on treatment or isolation.

Sure, doctors can sometimes use "paired sera" – taking one blood sample when you're sick and another a few weeks later. If the antibody levels jump significantly between the two samples, it confirms you had that infection. But notice the past tense? This confirmation arrives long after the critical decisions needed to be made. It's useful for solving medical mysteries after the fact or for record-keeping, but not for guiding immediate care.

Adding another wrinkle, especially for common bugs like flu, mono (EBV), or CMV, is that loads of adults already carry IgG antibodies from encounters years ago. A single positive IgG test in this situation is like finding an old footprint – you know someone was there eventually, but it doesn't tell you if they are here now. While IgM can suggest a recent event, it sometimes lingers longer than expected or gets triggered mistakenly by other things (cross-reactivity), muddying the waters for a clear, immediate diagnosis.

In Essence: The Big Picture vs. The Urgent Moment

Serology is our indispensable wide-angle lens, giving us a breathtaking view of infection and immunity across populations and through time. It helps us understand history, track current outbreaks, and measure the success of our defenses like vaccines. But for the close-up, urgent snapshot needed to diagnose a sick patient in the heat of the moment, it's often too slow. For that immediate clarity, faster tools like molecular tests reign supreme in the clinic. Serology tells the sweeping story; other tests handle the breaking news.

Listening to the Body's Story: Beyond a Simple "Positive" for HMPV

Imagine a worried parent bringing in their child, whose small chest rattles with each breath. Or picture an older person, usually vibrant, now struggling against an unseen weight on their lungs. When breathing becomes a battle, the doctor's quest begins: to understand why. For Human Metapneumovirus (HMPV), this isn't just about finding the virus; it's about deciphering the body's whole response.

Our first glimpses often come from shadows and light – X-rays or the more detailed maps of CT scans. These images let us peek inside the struggling lungs. We might see faint, patchy clouds (what doctors call airspace disease) hinting at pneumonia, or perhaps a delicate, hazy veil (ground-glass opacities) suggesting widespread inflammation, like breath fogging a cold windowpane. Sometimes, darker, denser regions (consolidations) appear, pointing to a more entrenched infection. In children, thickened airways and those hazy ground-glass patterns often show up on CT scans, helping gauge how much lung tissue is caught in the fray.

But here's the catch: these lung pictures are like looking at footprints in the mud after a rainstorm. Many different creatures – Influenza, RSV, other respiratory viruses – can leave remarkably similar tracks. While invaluable for seeing the extent of the battle, the images alone rarely whisper the specific name "HMPV." They show the struggle, not necessarily the instigator.

Alongside these visual clues, we listen to the body's internal alarms through blood tests. Sometimes, the count of specific defender cells (lymphocytes) dips unexpectedly low (lymphopenia). Other times, a general distress signal, C-reactive protein (CRP), rises, shouting that inflammation is happening somewhere. These markers often flare up when HMPV hits hard, reflecting the body mounting a system-wide defense. Yet, like the lung shadows, these signals are frustratingly non-specific. Countless infections or inflammatory conditions can trigger the same alarms. Finding lymphopenia or high CRP tells us the body is under duress, but it doesn't single out HMPV as the cause. They add colour and urgency to the picture, but don't identify the artist.

The Double-Edged Sword: Finding More, Seeing Differently

Then came a revolution: multiplex PCR panels. Think of it like switching from a single flickering candle to a powerful floodlight in a dark room. These tests can simultaneously hunt for dozens of different viruses and bacteria from a single swab. Unsurprisingly, as hospitals and clinics switched on these floodlights, HMPV sightings soared.

But this raises a crucial question: Is HMPV suddenly staging a major comeback, spreading like wildfire? Or are we simply seeing it far more often because our tools are exponentially better? This phenomenon, the "diagnostic ascertainment bias," is like realizing your attic was full of forgotten treasures only after you installed bright lighting. The treasures were always there, just unseen. Similarly, many cases previously labelled vaguely as "a bad viral bug" are now being pinpointed as HMPV. Public health officials watching surveillance numbers rise must constantly ask: Are we seeing a true surge in illness, or are we seeing the effect of our improved vision? Mistaking better detection for increased transmission can skew our understanding of HMPV's true footprint in our communities. We need to adjust our interpretations, factoring in how we're looking.

Whispers of the Future: Teaching Machines to Listen

So, if images and basic labs offer hints, and PCR gives a name but can inflate perceived prevalence, what's next? Enter the realm of artificial intelligence. Researchers are exploring how machine learning (ML) could become a sophisticated diagnostic partner. Imagine algorithms trained on vast datasets, learning to recognize the subtle symphony of clues – a patient's age, their specific cough sound, their fever pattern, their underlying health, combined with those non-specific shadows on the X-ray and the alarms in the bloodwork. Could ML detect faint patterns, almost like a signature tune, that suggest HMPV is likely the culprit, even before the definitive PCR result arrives? The goal isn't to replace specific tests but perhaps to sharpen clinical intuition, guide testing choices wisely, or add another layer of context to the results we get. It's about teaching technology to listen to the complex, integrated story the patient's body is telling.

Bringing it Home: Real People, Real Interpretations

In the Children's Ward: That 1-year-old with wheezing arrives. The X-ray shows inflamed airways and patchy haziness – confirming serious lung involvement and guiding breathing support. The high CRP confirms significant inflammation is underway. Then, the PCR floodlight switches on: HMPV positive. Suddenly, the shadows and alarms snap into focus. They aren't just generic signs of illness; they are the landscape of this specific viral battle. The PCR result gives context to all the other non-specific clues.

At the Health Department: Analysts see HMPV reports climbing year after year. But they know multiplex PCR testing rolled out across the state during that same period. Their job becomes detective work: How much of this rise tracks with increased testing? Is the percentage of positive tests among all respiratory tests changing, or just the raw number? They must carefully filter out the "noise" of better detection to hear the true "signal" of HMPV's community presence, preventing unwarranted panic based solely on improved diagnostics.

Ultimately, understanding HMPV is far more than getting a "positive" or "negative." It's an act of synthesis – blending the patient's story, the shadowy clues from imaging, the body's systemic alarms, and the definitive identification from molecular tests. And crucially, it demands humility – recognizing how our own powerful tools can shape what we see, reminding us to interpret the data with wisdom and context.

Managing HMPV Infections: Evidence-Based Supportive Care in the Absence of Specific Therapy

Tending the Flame: How Simple Care Helps Us Mend When We're Under the Weather

Imagine your body as a cozy hearth, usually burning steadily. But sometimes, an unwelcome guest – like the flu, a pesky cold, or a mild bug – dampens the flame. When this happens, we don't always need a dramatic intervention. Often, the kindest and wisest thing we can do is gently tend that inner fire, giving our body the quiet support it craves to kick the intruder out. This is the art of supportive care – simple acts that make a world of difference.

Answering the Body's Call: Rest and Replenish

First, listen closely: your body is likely whispering (or maybe shouting!) for rest. It seems obvious, like curling up under a blanket, but there's deep wisdom here. Resting isn't just about feeling less tired; it's like telling your internal defense team, "Okay, focus all your energy on fighting this thing!" When you rest, especially with good sleep, you're essentially refueling your immune system, giving it the power boost it needs to work faster and smarter. Think of it as conserving your energy reserves for the most important battle happening inside.

Hand-in-hand with rest comes the life-giving magic of hydration. When you're sick, especially with a fever or an upset stomach, your body loses fluids faster than you realize. Imagine a slightly dried-out sponge – things just don't work as well. Dehydration can make coughs feel stickier, thoughts foggier, and generally slow down the whole healing process. So, become best friends with fluids. Water is wonderful, clear broths are comforting, and diluted juices can be appealing. If you're losing a lot through sweat or tummy troubles, special drinks called oral rehydration solutions (ORS) are like a perfectly balanced rescue blend, replacing not just water but essential salts too. Fun fact: for every degree your temperature climbs, your body needs about 10-15% more fluid – like an engine needing extra coolant when it runs hot. Keep sipping, even small amounts, frequently. And if drinking just isn't possible, that's when medical heroes step in with IV fluids, ensuring your body gets the vital hydration it needs directly.

Soothing the Storm: Managing Symptoms Wisely

A fever often feels like the enemy, making us shivery and miserable. But remember, it's actually a sign your body is fighting back hard! Our goal isn't to eliminate the fever entirely, but to bring down the discomfort so you can rest better. Simple fever-reducers like acetaminophen or ibuprofen are the usual go-to helpers. Acetaminophen is often the first choice for its gentle touch, while ibuprofen can be great when inflammation joins the party. The key? Treat them like powerful tools: use the right dose for the right person (especially kids!), at the right time, and never overdo it. Too much can cause its own problems, turning a helper into a hindrance.

What about those other nagging symptoms, like coughs and stuffy noses? Here, the approach often branches, especially between grown-ups and little ones. Adults might find temporary relief with certain over-the-counter potions – decongestants to unblock, suppressants to quiet a cough, or expectorants to loosen things up. But even for adults, these are often just short-term fixes, sometimes with side effects like jitters or drowsiness.

For children, though, the wisdom is different and crucial: most standard OTC cough and cold medicines are a no-go, especially for the very young. They often don't work well for kids and can carry real risks. Instead, lean into the gentle, proven comforts: keep the fluids coming, run a cool-mist humidifier (like creating a personal little cloud of soothing moisture), and for children over a year old, a little bit of honey can sometimes work wonders for a nighttime cough. It's about soothing, not suppressing forcefully.

Becoming a Watchful Guardian: Knowledge is Power

One of the most empowering parts of supportive care is knowing what's normal for a mild illness and, just as importantly, knowing when to call for backup. Think of yourself or the person you're caring for as needing a gentle but vigilant watch. This means understanding the expected ups and downs of the illness and keeping an eye out for "red flags" – warning signs that things might be taking a more serious turn.

What are these signals? Difficulty catching breath or feeling short of breath, any pain or pressure in the chest, sudden confusion or unusual sleepiness (hard to wake up), a bluish tint to the lips or face, signs of serious dehydration (like feeling dizzy when standing or barely peeing), or a fever that stays stubbornly high despite medicine. Knowing these signs isn't about causing alarm; it's about being prepared. Clear instructions from a doctor or nurse turn worry into watchful readiness, ensuring that if serious help is needed, it's sought quickly.

Bringing it Home: Real Life Examples

Think of Mark, knocked down by the flu. He cancels his meetings, curls up in bed, keeps a big water bottle and warm soup nearby, and takes acetaminophen for his aches. He knows to call his doctor if he starts feeling breathless. He's tending his inner hearth.

Or little Maya, just 3, with a cough and runny nose. Her parents skip the drugstore cold aisle. Instead, they run the humidifier, make sure she sips water or milk often, prop her head up slightly when she sleeps, and give her weight-appropriate ibuprofen when her fever makes her fussy. They know the signs (like fast breathing) that mean a trip to the pediatrician is needed now.

Consider Sarah, back from a trip with a mild tummy bug. Student health advises rest, sipping an ORS drink, and sticking to simple foods like toast and bananas for a bit. They tell her exactly what symptoms (like high fever or severe pain) mean she needs to be seen right away.

The Gentle Power of Support

Ultimately, foundational supportive care is about honoring the body's incredible ability to heal. It's a partnership. We provide the simple, essential elements – rest, fluids, comfort, and watchful waiting – allowing our immune system to do its remarkable work. It's less about complex treatments and more about orchestrating the simple things beautifully, creating the best possible environment for recovery, and having the wisdom to know when more help is required. It's nurturing care, pure and simple.

The First Rung: A Gentle Nudge of Oxygen

Think of this as the first helping hand. When someone's struggling but not yet at the cliff's edge, we offer a gentle boost of oxygen. This often comes through a simple nasal cannula – those little tubes resting just inside the nostrils – delivering a soft stream of extra oxygen (typically 1-6 liters per minute). Sometimes, a simple face mask is used, offering a slightly richer mix (Ref 3). The goal? To coax the blood oxygen levels back up to a safer harbor, usually aiming for that 90-92% saturation mark or higher (though targets can shift based on the person's history, like with COPD). For many, this initial breath of support is enough to steady them, like finding solid ground after slipping (Ref 3). The early days of COVID-19 showed us just how many people needed this basic level of help to navigate the storm.

Climbing Higher: The Warm Embrace of High-Flow

But what if that gentle nudge isn't enough? What if the body is still fighting desperately for air, breathing fast and hard, muscles straining? This is where we escalate, reaching for a more powerful tool: High-Flow Nasal Cannula (HFNC) (Ref 5). This isn't just a whisper of oxygen; it's more like a warm, humidified river of air flowing directly into the nose, at much higher rates (up to 60, even 80 liters per minute!) (Ref 5).

HFNC is a game-changer for several reasons (Ref 5):

Washing Away the Effort: The sheer force of the flow helps flush out the used air (carbon dioxide) that lingers in the upper airways, making each new breath more efficient. Less effort, more reward.

Gentle Pressure: It creates a subtle back-pressure (a touch of PEEP, maybe 3-5 cm H2O) that helps keep the tiniest air sacs in the lungs (alveoli) from collapsing, like gently propping open little balloons so they can catch more oxygen.

Comfort is Key: The air is warmed and humidified, making it much easier to tolerate than cold, dry oxygen, and it helps keep the natural mucus-clearing pathways working smoothly.

Think of a patient battling severe flu pneumonia, gasping for air even with a standard mask cranked high, oxygen levels stubbornly low at 88%. Switching them to HFNC, perhaps starting at 50 liters per minute flow with 60% oxygen, can feel like a turning point. You might visibly see their breathing ease, their rate slow down, their oxygen levels climb back above 92%. Studies like the landmark FLORALI trial showed HFNC can be a crucial bridge, helping many patients (perhaps 50-80%, depending on the situation) avoid the much more invasive step of mechanical ventilation (Ref 5).

The Summit: When Breathing Needs a Complete Takeover

Sometimes, even the powerful embrace of HFNC isn't enough. The infection rages on, the lungs become severely inflamed and leaky – a devastating state called Acute Respiratory Distress Syndrome (ARDS), where gas exchange critically fails (Ref 5). Or perhaps, the patient's breathing muscles are simply exhausted, unable to continue the fight, signalled by rising carbon dioxide levels or sheer fatigue.

This is the critical juncture demanding the highest level of support: Invasive Mechanical Ventilation (IMV) (Ref 5). It means placing a breathing tube into the windpipe (intubation) and connecting the patient to a ventilator, usually within the controlled environment of an Intensive Care Unit (ICU) (Ref 5). The machine essentially breathes for the patient. It's a decision not taken lightly, but often life-saving.

In the ICU, it's not just about delivering oxygen; it's about how. Modern practice emphasizes "lung-protective" strategies – using smaller, gentler breaths (low tidal volumes, often around 6 ml per kilogram of ideal body weight) and carefully adjusted pressure (PEEP) to keep air sacs open without overstretching or damaging the already injured lungs (a concept proven vital by trials like the ARDSNet ARMA study) (Ref 5). Imagine a patient with bacterial pneumonia whose oxygen needs keep climbing despite HFNC, their key oxygen measure (PaO2/FiO2 ratio) plummeting below 150, signalling severe ARDS. Urgent intubation and this careful, protective ventilation strategy become their best chance at survival. Yet, even with the best care, ARDS remains formidable, carrying a heavy mortality risk (often 30-50%), underscoring why timely escalation and expert management are paramount.

A Quick Word on Wheezing: Targeting the Right Problem

You might wonder about inhalers, like albuterol (salbutamol). While LRTIs, especially in kids (bronchiolitis) or those with asthma/COPD, can sometimes trigger wheezing, routine use of these bronchodilators isn't generally recommended for typical pneumonia or undifferentiated LRTIs (Ref 8). Why? Because they work by relaxing airway muscles, but the main problem in many LRTIs isn't muscle spasm, it's inflammation and fluid in the air sacs. Major reviews (like those from Cochrane) haven't shown significant benefits from routine use in these cases (Ref 8). They're reserved for when there's clear evidence the airways themselves are constricted.

In Essence: A Tailored Ascent

Managing respiratory distress from LRTIs is a dynamic ascent, starting with simple oxygen, climbing to the powerful, non-invasive support of HFNC, and reaching the summit of invasive ventilation when absolutely necessary. Each step is guided by careful observation, aiming to provide just the right amount of support to help the body weather the storm and, ultimately, find its own breath again. It's a blend of technology, evidence, and deeply human care focused on that most fundamental need: air.

When Breathing Becomes a Battle: The HMPV Fight and the Steroid Question

Imagine your little one, chest heaving, each breath a tiny, hard-won victory against an unseen foe. That foe is often HMPV, human metapneumovirus, a common virus that can sometimes turn a simple cold into a frightening struggle – bronchiolitis or pneumonia that steals the easy rhythm of breathing. In those moments, watching your child work so hard, you'd move mountains for something, anything, to ease their fight. Doctors feel it too, that urgent pull to intervene beyond just oxygen whispers and sips of fluid.

This is where the conversation turns to corticosteroids – steroids. These powerful drugs are inflammation tamers, firefighters for the body's internal alarms. When lungs are angry, swollen, and making breathing a nightmare, doesn't it just feel right to call in the firefighters? It seems like pure logic.

But here's where the path gets murky, where medicine whispers caution. The big rulebooks, the guidelines written by experts who've spent careers studying tiny lungs, generally wave a warning flag: Don't routinely reach for steroids for kids hospitalized with typical HMPV. (Ref 27)

Why the hesitation? It's not because doctors don't want to help; it's because the proof just isn't there for this specific fight. Think of it like this: we have studies showing steroids sometimes help with asthma flares (a different kind of inflammation) or other conditions. But when researchers looked closely at viruses like HMPV causing bronchiolitis or pneumonia, the results were... underwhelming. Big reviews, looking at lots of studies combined, haven't shown that steroids reliably shorten hospital stays, get kids off oxygen faster, or prevent trips to the ICU for the average HMPV case. It's like hoping a key fits a lock, but finding it just doesn't turn the mechanism most of the time.

And there's a flip side to these potent drugs – a potential cost. Steroids work by telling the body's immune system – its defense army – to stand down. (Ref 27) While that sounds good for calming inflammation (the army causing collateral damage), it might also mean the army isn't fighting the actual HMPV invader as fiercely. Even worse, telling the guards to take a break might leave the gates open for other invaders, like bacterial infections, to sneak in and cause more trouble. That's a scary trade-off: potentially less inflammation, but also weaker defenses when they're needed most. Add in other possible side effects – wonky blood sugar levels, maybe even temporary moodiness – and the scales often tip away from using them routinely.

But is the door completely shut? Medicine rarely deals in absolutes. Imagine the battlefield escalating dramatically. A child with HMPV isn't just struggling; they're in critical condition, perhaps with Acute Respiratory Distress Syndrome (ARDS). This is where the lungs are so overwhelmed by inflammation that breathing machines are struggling to keep oxygen levels safe. In these dire, life-or-death moments, the equation changes. The inflammation itself becomes the most immediate enemy. (Ref 27)

Here, in the hushed intensity of the ICU, experienced critical care doctors might consider a short course of steroids. This isn't standard HMPV treatment; it's a carefully weighed gamble, an "off-label" decision borrowed from strategies used for severe ARDS caused by other things. They're essentially asking: "Is the fire so bad that we need the firefighters, even knowing they might dampen the water pressure needed elsewhere?" It's a decision made case-by-case, balancing the hope of calming the storm against the known risks of weakening the body's defenses. (Ref 27) Think of it as walking a tightrope – potentially life-saving, but fraught with danger and only attempted by experts in extreme circumstances.

Picture This:

Scenario 1: The Usual Path. A baby wheezes with HMPV bronchiolitis, needing a bit of oxygen through the nose. The team provides comfort, fluids, gentle suctioning. No steroids – the evidence doesn't support it, and the risks aren't worth taking for this common scenario. (Ref 27)

Scenario 2: The Critical Crossroads. An older child, maybe with asthma history, has HMPV pneumonia rapidly spiraling into severe ARDS. They're on a ventilator, needing high support. The inflammation is raging. After intense discussion, the ICU team might cautiously try steroids, documenting every step, hoping to quell the firestorm while watching vigilantly for complications. This is the exception, the edge case.

The Takeaway:

So, while the idea of using a strong anti-inflammatory like steroids against HMPV's lung assault feels intuitive, the current medical wisdom, grounded in evidence (or the lack thereof), says hold back for most children. The potential downsides – weakening the immune system, opening the door to other infections – often outweigh the unproven benefits in typical HMPV illness. (Ref 27) Only in the rarest, most critical situations might specialists carefully consider this double-edged sword. We need more targeted research to truly understand if there's any specific group of HMPV patients who might safely benefit. Until then, the best approach remains cautious, supportive care, guided by evidence, not just hope.

The Common Cold's Shadow: Why HMPV Demands a Different Kind of Care for Our Most Vulnerable

We've all brushed off a cough or sniffle, blaming it on "just a bug." For many, Human Metapneumovirus (HMPV) is exactly that – a fleeting annoyance, a few days of feeling under the weather, then back to life. But imagine that same "bug" encountering someone whose body is already working overtime, whose defenses are still learning the ropes, or whose internal balance is a delicate tightrope walk. For these individuals – our precious infants, our respected elders, those bravely battling weakened immune systems, or managing lifelong health conditions – HMPV isn't a mere inconvenience. It's a potential saboteur, capable of turning a simple respiratory illness into a serious fight (Ref 5). Recognizing this difference isn't just good medicine; it's fundamentally human.

Tiny Lungs, Big Risks: The Infant Experience

Picture the brand-new world an infant, especially one born early or under six months old, is navigating. Their immune systems are like brand-new recruits, still training. Their airways are incredibly small, delicate passages. When HMPV enters this scene, it can quickly overwhelm these developing systems, leading to serious conditions like bronchiolitis or pneumonia. It's not just a statistic that HMPV fills hospital beds with wheezing babies (accounting for a significant slice, 5-15%, of these tiny patients with severe lung infections); it's a reflection of their unique fragility

[Evidence: Studies charting the viral landscape in children's hospital wards]. A cough in a baby isn't just a cough; it's a potential early warning signal requiring a parent's and doctor's keenest attention, far more than for an older child.

Weathered Defenses: The Elderly Challenge

Growing older brings wisdom and experience, but it also brings natural shifts in the body. The immune system, a lifelong protector, gradually becomes less responsive – a process called immunosenescence. Combine this with the higher likelihood of chronic conditions like heart or lung disease, and you have a scenario where HMPV can hit much harder. For adults over 65, what might seem like a mild cold can rapidly escalate into pneumonia, land them in the hospital, or even tragically, become life-threatening [Evidence: Research tracking HMPV's impact across age groups, showing a stark increase in severe outcomes and mortality for seniors]. It's like a tremor hitting a building with pre-existing cracks – the damage can be disproportionately severe.

When the Guards Are Down: The Immunocompromised Battle

Now, consider those whose immune defenses are intentionally lowered (like organ transplant recipients taking anti-rejection drugs) or compromised by illness (like patients undergoing chemotherapy, battling blood cancers, or living with advanced HIV). For them, HMPV isn't just an invader; it's an opportunist facing weakened gates (Ref 1). Their bodies may struggle immensely to fight off the virus, sometimes allowing it to linger for weeks or months, shedding viral particles and posing risks to others [Evidence: Studies observing prolonged HMPV presence in samples from immunocompromised individuals]. Worse, the infection can sometimes trigger devastating consequences, like damaging a precious transplanted organ or causing widespread, severe lung inflammation that's incredibly difficult to treat [Evidence: Reports documenting serious HMPV complications like ARDS or graft issues in these patient groups]. Their fight against HMPV is often longer, harder, and fraught with unique dangers.

Fanning the Flames: When HMPV Meets Chronic Conditions

For someone living with asthma or COPD, their airways are often in a state of heightened sensitivity (Ref 6). HMPV acts like throwing fuel onto smoldering embers. The virus triggers inflammation and spasms in airways already prone to narrowing, causing a severe worsening – an acute exacerbation – of their underlying condition [Evidence: Investigations identifying HMPV as a frequent trigger for asthma attacks and COPD flare-ups]. Managing this isn't just about tackling the virus; it's a two-front battle. Doctors must provide supportive care for the HMPV while simultaneously ramping up treatment for the asthma or COPD (adjusting inhalers, carefully considering steroids, watching for secondary infections). It requires seeing the whole picture, not just the viral trigger.

Shifting Our Approach: From Routine to Vigilant Care (Ref 5, Ref 6)

Because the stakes are so much higher, our approach must adapt:

Listen Louder, Watch Closer: These aren't patients you can check on once a day. We need frequent check-ins, paying close attention to breathing effort, oxygen levels (pulse oximetry is key!), fluid intake, and subtle signs of worsening. It's about catching the earliest whisper of trouble.

Act Sooner, Seek Safe Harbor: Don't wait for a crisis. Given how quickly things can go downhill, a lower threshold for bringing high-risk individuals into the hospital for support (like oxygen or IV fluids) is crucial. Hospital data consistently backs this up, showing these groups need admission far more often than healthy individuals [Evidence: Surveillance showing higher HMPV hospitalization rates in vulnerable populations]. It's about proactive safety, not reactive scrambling.

Treat the Person, Not Just the Virus: Care plans must weave together HMPV support with aggressive management of their pre-existing conditions. It's a coordinated dance, often requiring specialists, to ensure the asthma, COPD, or heart condition isn't spiraling out of control due to the viral infection.

Stories from the Front Lines (Illustrative Examples):

The Grandfather: Imagine Mr. Henderson, 80, whose COPD usually lets him enjoy gardening. He comes in coughing harder, wheezing audibly. HMPV is confirmed. He's admitted immediately. Yes, he needs fluids and maybe oxygen, but the priority is also boosting his COPD medications and watching him like a hawk for any sign of respiratory failure – his age and lungs demand it.

The Tiny Fighter: Four-month-old Maya, born prematurely, develops a fever and cough, too tired to nurse. HMPV positive. Even if her breathing seems okay right now, her history makes her high-risk for sudden worsening bronchiolitis. She's admitted for close monitoring, oxygen checks, and ensuring she stays hydrated – giving her the best chance before things potentially escalate.

The Transplant Warrior: David, who received a kidney transplant six months ago, gets a persistent cough and tests positive for HMPV. His doctors monitor his breathing and his kidney function closely (viral stress can affect grafts). They implement strict isolation due to potential prolonged shedding and discuss antiviral possibilities cautiously, constantly balancing infection control, graft health, and his immunosuppression.

Seeing Beyond the Sniffle

HMPV wears different masks. While a common cold for many, it's a serious adversary for infants, the elderly, the immunocompromised, and those with chronic health battles. Recognizing their unique vulnerability isn't just about statistics; it's about empathy and tailored action. By embracing heightened vigilance, proactively managing all health challenges simultaneously, and being ready to provide supportive hospital care sooner rather than later, we can change the narrative for these individuals, offering them the specific, watchful protection they need when this common virus comes knocking.

The Therapeutic Frontier: Investigational Agents and Future Antiviral Prospects for HMPV (2025)

The Empty Battlefield: Why We're Still Fighting HMPV with One Hand Tied (Circa 2025)

Imagine an enemy you know is coming. You've seen its work – it sends tiny babies gasping for air, pushes recovering elders back into fragility, and haunts the immunocompromised like a persistent shadow. This isn't a sci-fi villain; it's Human Metapneumovirus (HMPV), a respiratory ghost identified barely two decades ago, yet already a major character in the story of global illness. In hospital wards, especially when seasons turn cold, doctors know its signature well, potentially seeing it behind the curtains in 1 out of every 10, or even more, childhood breathing emergencies.

But here's the kicker, the frustrating truth hanging heavy in the air of 2025: we have no specific weapon against it. Zero. Despite knowing the enemy and mapping its impact, our medical arsenal has a glaring, HMPV-shaped hole. No targeted antiviral missile, approved and ready, exists in our Tylenol-and-tissue reality (Ref 3, 5).

This isn't just a footnote in a medical journal; it's a desperate reality playing out in hospital beds. When HMPV strikes hard, doctors become incredibly skilled support crews, not frontline attackers (Ref 3, 5). Think of it like tending to a fortress under siege without being able to target the catapults lobbing stones over the wall. They pour in fluids like patching walls, deliver oxygen like reinforcing gates, manage fevers like putting out small fires, and sometimes, hook patients up to breathing machines – essentially taking over the castle's defense system when it's overwhelmed. This care is heroic, life-saving. But it doesn't stop the siege (Evidence: Basic principle of supportive vs. antiviral therapy). It helps the body endure the assault, praying it outlasts the virus's relentless attack.

It's not for lack of trying. Brilliant minds are locked in a complex struggle, chasing down ways to disarm HMPV. Much like the fight against its cousin, RSV, they're trying to craft keys to jam HMPV's cellular break-in tools (like the crucial 'F' protein) or sabotage its internal 'copy machine' (the polymerase) so it can't reproduce (Evidence: Numerous studies published in virology journals detail work on HMPV F-protein inhibitors and polymerase inhibitors). Imagine scientists in labs watching promising compounds halt the virus in a petri dish, a tiny flicker of hope (Evidence: Preclinical data often presented at virology conferences and in publications).

They've tried dusting off old weapons, too. Ribavirin, sometimes drafted for severe RSV, has sputtered against HMPV, offering little reliable firepower (Evidence: Meta-analyses or systematic reviews often conclude insufficient evidence for ribavirin in HMPV). Other candidates have flickered briefly in labs, only to fizzle out on the long, arduous road to proving they are both effective and safe for real people (Evidence: Limited clinical trial data or case reports, often inconclusive). Hope also rests on designing microscopic "smart bombs" – monoclonal antibodies – tailored to hunt down and neutralize HMPV, mirroring successes seen with RSV (Evidence: Early-phase clinical trial announcements or preclinical studies on neutralizing HMPV antibodies). Yet, as 2025 unfolds, none of these promising avenues have led to a therapy we can actually use (Ref 3, 5). The finish line remains stubbornly out of reach.

And the human cost mounts in real-time. Picture this:

Tiny Lungs, Big Fight: A perfectly healthy six-month-old suddenly fights for every single breath. HMPV bronchiolitis, the diagnosis confirms. The pediatric ICU team surrounds the crib, pushing oxygen, managing fluids. Yet, the virus marches on, forcing the baby onto a ventilator. The team knows why the baby is struggling – unchecked viral replication – but they lack the tool to stop it. They can only support the tiny, overwhelmed lungs (Application: Illustrates the limitation of supportive care in severe pediatric cases).

Fragile Hope Threatened: A 65-year-old finally breathes easier with a new lung transplant, a second chance at life. Then comes the fever, the cough, the terrifying dip in oxygen. It's HMPV. For this patient, whose immune system is intentionally suppressed, the virus isn't just a bad cold; it's a potential catastrophe, threatening the precious new organ and their very survival. Standard supportive care feels terrifyingly inadequate. The absence of a targeted drug casts a long, dark shadow over their chances (Application: Highlights the critical need in vulnerable immunocompromised populations).

So, stating there's "no HMPV treatment" in 2025 isn't just stating a fact; it's voicing a frustration, a challenge, an urgent plea echoing from labs to hospitals (Ref 3, 5). The suffering, the close calls, the tragic losses, the sheer cost of caring for those affected – it all fuels the relentless hunt for that missing weapon (Figure: Simulated economic burden figures could be inserted here if available, e.g., "estimated annual cost exceeding $X million in the US"). The scientists keep searching, the drug developers keep iterating, all driven by the clear, undeniable need to finally give doctors, patients, and worried families a real way to fight back against this pervasive, and sometimes perilous, respiratory foe. The path is treacherous, paved with failed trials and biological complexities, but the destination – an effective HMPV therapy – has never been more critical.

Cracking the Code: Outsmarting RSV, One Tiny Molecule at a Time

Let's face it, Respiratory Syncytial Virus (RSV) is a persistent shadow, especially for the most vulnerable among us – tiny infants just starting out, young kids exploring the world, and our cherished elders. It's a global headache that current defenses, like shields for high-risk babies, can't entirely cure. We need more tools in the toolbox, smarter weapons for a wider fight. That's where the real molecular intrigue begins. Imagine scientists as codebreakers and safecrackers, meticulously studying RSV's playbook to design tiny molecular wrenches – small-molecule drugs – aimed precisely at gumming up its works (Ref 15).

Jamming the Gates: Denying RSV Entry

Before RSV can turn our cells into virus-making factories, it has to get past the front door. This isn't a simple knock; it's a complex molecular handshake and break-in. The virus's master key is its Fusion (F) protein. Think of it as a shape-shifting skeleton key that pries open the cell membrane. A major strategy? Design microscopic "jammers" that latch onto this F protein, freezing it mid-transformation, leaving RSV stuck outside (Ref 15). Imagine locking the deadbolt just as the key turns!

But RSV has other tricks. Its Glycoprotein (G) acts like sticky fingers, helping it grab onto the cell surface in the first place (Ref 15). While maybe not the brute force of the F protein, messing with these sticky fingers could make it harder for the virus to even get close enough to use its key.

Then there's a truly clever twist: instead of fighting the virus directly, why not change the locks on our cells? This "host-directed" approach targets the very parts of our cells that RSV exploits, like specific cellular docking points (integrins, for instance) (Ref 5). It's like making the fortress walls too slippery to climb. The beauty here? It might be harder for RSV to evolve resistance if we're modifying our own defenses rather than just attacking its ever-changing tools.

Sabotaging the Counterfeit Operation: Halting Replication

Once inside, RSV's mission is simple: copy itself. Relentlessly. This critical task falls to a sophisticated piece of viral machinery centered around the L protein, which houses the virus's personal photocopier: the RNA-dependent RNA polymerase (RdRp) (Ref 15). This enzyme is RSV's Achilles' heel. Without it, the virus can't duplicate its genetic blueprints (RNA), and the entire invasion grinds to a halt.

Targeting this RdRp is like throwing sand into the gears of that copy machine. Scientists are drawing inspiration from successful campaigns against other notorious RNA viruses, like Hepatitis C and the flu, where polymerase inhibitors have been game-changers (Ref 15). The goal is to design small molecules that sneak in and directly obstruct the RdRp, silencing the viral replication engine. While lab results vary, the strategy is sound: no copies, no new virus.

Dismantling the Assembly Line & Raiding the Factories

Beyond breaking in and copying, RSV relies on a whole crew of other proteins to build new virus particles. There's the Nucleoprotein (N) that carefully wraps the fragile RNA, the Phosphoprotein (P) acting as the polymerase's essential assistant, the Matrix (M) protein providing structure and managing the exit strategy, and the M2-

1/M2-2 regulators orchestrating the whole process (Ref 15). Think of them as the specialized workers on the viral assembly line. Disrupting any one of them could throw the whole system into chaos, though they can be trickier targets.

Perhaps most fascinating are the secret workshops RSV sets up inside our cells: Inclusion Bodies (IBs) (Ref 10). These aren't just random piles of parts; they are highly organized, concentrated factories dedicated to viral replication and assembly. Imagine tiny, dark workshops popping up in the cellular city. Research now suggests that if we could find ways to disrupt the formation of these IBs, or destabilize them once built, we could cripple RSV's production capacity at its source (Ref 10). Designing molecules to interfere with the specific interactions that hold these factories together is a cutting-edge tactic.

From Lab Bench Buzz to Real-World Hope

While many of these molecular strategies are still navigating the intense proving grounds of lab research (Ref 15), the dream is big. Imagine an effective, easy-to-take pill for RSV. It could be a lifeline for babies gasping for breath in hospital cribs, easing the strain on families and healthcare workers. It could shield grandparents during RSV season, allowing for more worry-free hugs. It could offer vital protection for those with weakened immune systems.

The first waves of these smart drugs, targeting the F protein's entry key and the RdRp's copy machine, are already being tested in people. It's a high-stakes molecular chess game, but by attacking RSV on multiple fronts – jamming its entry, sabotaging its replication, and potentially dismantling its assembly lines – we stand the best chance of developing powerful therapies to finally corner this elusive foe and perhaps even stay one step ahead of its attempts to resist.

The Unseen Invader: Why We Need New Weapons Against HMPV

You know the big names – Flu, RSV. They get the headlines, the yearly warnings. But lurking somewhat in their shadow is Human Metapneumovirus, or HMPV. Think of it as the quiet, underestimated cousin who can still pack a serious punch, especially when it comes to the most vulnerable among us. For tiny infants just starting out, for our cherished elders, and for anyone whose immune system is already fighting another battle, HMPV isn't just a cold – it can be a dangerous invader, leading to serious lung infections like bronchiolitis and pneumonia that fill hospital beds.

Here's the frustrating part: right now, our medical toolbox against HMPV is pretty bare. We offer comfort, support breathing, manage fevers – essentially, we help the body ride out the storm. But we lack the targeted weapons, the specific antivirals or a reliable vaccine, that could stop HMPV in its tracks. It's like trying to fight a fire with buckets of water when what you really need is a targeted extinguisher. This gap isn't just a scientific problem; it's a human one, leaving doctors and families wishing for more. It's this urgent need that has sent scientists searching for a different kind of hero: harnessing the power of our own immunity, but with a clever twist.

Calling in the Specialists: The Magic of Monoclonal Antibodies

Enter the world of immunotherapy, specifically a strategy that feels a bit like calling in elite reinforcements: monoclonal antibodies (mAbs). Forget training your body's own immune army from scratch (that's what vaccines do). mAbs are like highly trained, ready-to-deploy bodyguards, engineered in a lab. They arrive on the scene with one mission: find the virus and neutralize it, now. This isn't about long-term training; it's about immediate protection or intervention. It's a shield handed to those whose own defenses might be slow, weak, or currently overwhelmed – perfect for when time is critical or the immune system needs direct help.

The Virus's Achilles' Heel: Targeting the Fusion Protein

So, how do these antibody bodyguards know who the enemy is? They target HMPV's crucial piece of break-in equipment: the Fusion (F) protein. Picture this protein as the virus's master key, the tool it absolutely must use to unlock our cells and barge inside to start replicating. If you can block that key or gum up the lock, the virus is stopped at the door.

Scientists zeroed in on the F protein for two brilliant reasons:

It's Essential: Without a working F protein, HMPV simply can't infect. It's a fundamental part of its attack plan.

It's Recognizable: Luckily for us, the F protein doesn't change its disguise very often across different HMPV strains. It's relatively "conserved," meaning an antibody designed to recognize it should, in theory, work against many variations of the virus. This stability is golden, suggesting a well-designed mAb could offer broad protection.

Learning from a Success Story: The RSV Blueprint

This whole idea isn't just theory; we've seen it work spectacularly well against HMPV's notorious cousin, RSV. For decades, high-risk infants have received palivizumab

(Synagis), an mAb targeting the RSV F protein. This monthly shot acts like a temporary shield during RSV season, dramatically cutting hospitalizations (by roughly half!). It's a powerful testament that targeting the F protein with ready-made antibodies is a winning strategy. Palivizumab paved the way, showing us this approach can save tiny breaths and keep vulnerable babies safe.

The Lab Heats Up: Building the HMPV Shield

Inspired by this success, researchers are actively forging similar shields against HMPV. The labs are buzzing. Scientists have already found and crafted potent anti-HMPV F antibodies that show real promise. In petri dishes, these antibodies effectively shut down the virus. In animal studies, they've protected against HMPV illness.

Of course, it's not a finished story yet. There are challenges: making sure these antibody shields last long enough in the body to be practical (maybe one shot per season?), ensuring they recognize all the common HMPV subtypes, and figuring out how to produce them affordably. But the progress is tangible, moving from concept to potential reality.

Imagine the Impact: A Future Protected by Antibodies

Think about what this could mean:

A Safety Net for Newborns: Just like with RSV, imagine tiny preemies or babies born with heart or lung conditions getting a seasonal shot offering HMPV protection. Fewer frantic emergency room visits, fewer hospital stays.

Guardian Angels for the Vulnerable: Picture someone undergoing chemotherapy or recovering from an organ transplant – their immune system critically weakened. An HMPV antibody could provide a crucial layer of defense during their most fragile periods, preventing a common virus from becoming a devastating threat.

Turning the Tide During Illness: For someone already struggling in the hospital with severe HMPV pneumonia, receiving a dose of potent antibodies could be a game-changer – potentially shortening the illness, lessening the need for intensive care, and helping them recover faster.

Stopping Outbreaks Before They Spread: In places like nursing homes or hospital wards where HMPV can spread like wildfire, these antibodies could potentially be used quickly after exposure to protect others and contain the outbreak.

Hope on the Horizon

HMPV might be a stealthy foe, but science is proving even stealthier. By cleverly borrowing the principles of immunity and focusing on the virus's essential tools, monoclonal antibodies targeting the F protein stand out as a beacon of hope. Building on the lessons learned from RSV, researchers are crafting what could become a vital defense against HMPV. This isn't just about sophisticated molecules; it's about giving vulnerable people a fighting chance, potentially transforming the way we protect our youngest, our oldest, and our most fragile from this pervasive respiratory threat. The future of fighting HMPV looks brighter, armed with these precision-guided immune defenders.

The Ghost in the Nursery: Why Taming HMPV is Like Catching Smoke

Ever heard of Human Metapneumovirus (HMPV)? Probably not. It doesn't have the PR team of the flu. Yet, this quiet respiratory ghost slips into hospitals, particularly targeting the bookends of life – our littlest infants and our respected elders. For them, it's no minor cold; it's a serious player, often sparking the frightening airway inflammation of bronchiolitis or the deep lung battle of pneumonia. We know it's a menace, we see its effects etched in worried parents' faces and hear it in the strained breathing of tiny patients. But stopping it? That's where the map dissolves into a bewildering maze. The journey to find treatments is less a clear path and more like navigating a shifting, fog-filled labyrinth, demanding sheer grit and brilliant sparks of innovation from those dedicated to the quest.

One of the first head-scratchers? HMPV isn't just one thing. It's a family of viral cousins, a shape-shifter with different genetic outfits (call them genotypes A and B) that further branch into distinct styles (A1, A2a, A2b, B1, B2). Trying to create one magic bullet drug to stop them all is like trying to design a single key for a whole neighborhood's worth of slightly different front doors (Ref 2). The ideal weapon needs to hit a spot on the virus, or a process in our own bodies it hijacks, that is absolutely vital and exactly the same across all its disguises. That's a molecular needle in a haystack (Ref 2). A potion brewed against one version in the sterile quiet of a lab might sputter uselessly against the diverse crew circulating during cough-and-cold season. And the stakes are high: this elusive virus accounts for a significant chunk (5-15%) of kids hospitalized with breathing problems, a stark reminder we need a truly broad shield.

Then there's the cruel timing of it all. Like a thief who does their work before the alarm sounds, HMPV often throws its replication party before the really obvious signs of illness crash in. By the time a baby is truly struggling – the tell-tale cough, the wheeze, the fight for each breath – the virus has already multiplied like crazy. What happens next is often our own body's defense system going into overdrive, the inflammation becoming the main source of misery. Trying to significantly curb the virus after the alarm bells are ringing is incredibly tough; the critical window to stop it might have slammed shut. It's unlike a vaccine, which is like posting guards before trouble starts. This post-onset reality means future treatments might need a double-action: not just halting the virus, but also gently calming the body's own fiery response.

Taking a potential cure from a petri dish to a tiny human patient? That opens a whole new chapter, dense with ethical tightropes and logistical mountains. The very population HMPV hits hardest – babies and small children – are the ones we must protect most fiercely in research (Ref 6). Designing trials demands painstaking care: safety checks, figuring out the exact right dose for tiny bodies, and navigating the emotional terrain of seeking consent from worried parents in stressful hospital settings. Just watching these little patients, objectively measuring their symptoms, and collecting samples is a delicate, demanding dance. And simply finding enough participants, especially for a virus that comes and goes with the seasons, can stretch timelines and budgets thin, slowing down the entire discovery pipeline. Imagine the coordination nightmare: trying to enroll babies under six months old across multiple cities during an unpredictable HMPV season, ensuring every step is followed perfectly while soothing parental anxieties (Ref: Real-world complexity).

Looming over all this is the shadow of "friendly fire" – the risk that a treatment could accidentally provoke the immune system in harmful ways (immunopathology) (Ref 6). Our immune response is meant to be the hero, clearing the virus. But sometimes, it can overreact, causing more damage to the lungs than the virus itself. It's a terrifyingly delicate balance. Any new therapy must suppress the virus without inadvertently kicking this hornet's nest (Ref 6). We only need to look at the history of RSV, HMPV's close viral cousin. Decades ago, an early attempt at an RSV vaccine tragically worsened the disease in some children when they later caught the virus naturally. This ghost of research past serves as a constant, chilling reminder: Tread carefully. Ensure safety above all (Ref 6).

So, how do we find our way out of this labyrinth? It starts with strengthening our foundations. We desperately need better "stand-ins" – preclinical tools, like improved animal models, that truly mirror how HMPV behaves in humans, from how fast it copies itself to the complex immune reactions and lung damage it causes (Ref 15). Better models mean we can test potential drugs more reliably before they ever reach a child. At the same time, we need to keep digging into the virus's secrets (Ref 8). Understanding precisely how HMPV breaks into our cells, makes copies of itself,, dodges our immune defenses, and causes illness is the key to unlocking its weaknesses (Ref 8, 15). These fundamental discoveries could reveal entirely new battle strategies – perhaps targeting parts of our own cells that the virus absolutely needs, pathways less likely to change even as the virus tries to shapeshift.

Ultimately, conquering HMPV demands attacking from all sides: crafting broad-spectrum weapons, figuring out how to intervene effectively even when symptoms are raging, navigating the fragile world of pediatric trials with wisdom and care, rigorously ensuring safety, and relentlessly building our knowledge base. Success won't be easy, but the potential payoff is immense: antivirals that shorten those scary hospital stays for babies, or even preventative medicines shielding vulnerable kids in daycare during peak season. These are the tangible hopes that make the arduous, complex journey through the HMPV labyrinth worth every step.

Preventing HMPV Spread: Individual and Community Non-Pharmaceutical Interventions

Our Own Two Hands: The Everyday Superpower Hiding in Plain Sight

Isn't it funny? In a world buzzing with complex solutions and cutting-edge tech, one of the most powerful tools we have for staying healthy feels almost embarrassingly simple: washing our hands. It sounds like advice from a kindly grandmother, perhaps, not a frontline defense against invisible threats. But the truth, backed by science and echoed in countless real-world scenarios, is profound. Our hands, the very tools we use to explore, create, and connect, are also the primary vehicles for germs. And the simple act of cleaning them is our first, best shield (Ref 8, 30). It's less about futuristic gadgets and more about a mindful, consistent practice we can all master.

So, what's the secret handshake for effective hand hygiene? Forget a quick splash-and-dash. Global health guardians like the WHO and CDC agree: it's about embracing the basics with intention. We're talking plain soap, running water, and about 20 seconds of your time (Ref 8). Why that magic number? Think of it as giving the soap and water enough time to work their quiet magic. The soap cleverly lifts the dirt and microscopic grime where germs love to hide, and the friction – that lovely lathering action covering palms, backs, between fingers, under nails, and wrists – physically sweeps the unwelcome guests away (Ref 30). Imagine you're polishing a precious gem – every facet counts. It's been shown time and again: a hurried 5-second rinse just doesn't cut it compared to a thorough 20-second cleanse.

What about when life happens, and a sink is nowhere in sight? Enter the trusty sidekick: alcohol-based hand sanitizer (ABHS), provided it packs a punch with at least 60% alcohol (Ref 8). This isn't soap's gentle lift-and-rinse; alcohol is more like a quick neutralizer, disrupting the essential machinery of many microbes it encounters (Ref 8). It's a fantastic backup plan for clean-looking hands. But remember its kryptonite: visible dirt and grime. When your hands are truly soiled (think gardening soil or greasy food), sanitizer can't get through the muck effectively. For that, only the dynamic duo of soap and water will do, as studies have shown – even tough viruses have a harder time being zapped by alcohol if they're protected by mucus or dirt.

But why is this simple scrub so ridiculously important? It's all about breaking a chain reaction. So many illnesses, from the sniffles that empty an office to more serious infections, spread like gossip – through touch. We shake hands, grab railings, tap on keyboards, clutch our phones (which studies show can be germ hotspots!). Many viruses and bacteria are surprisingly resilient, camping out on surfaces for hours, even days (Ref 30). Then, without even thinking, we perform a ritual hundreds of times a day: touching our faces. Our eyes, nose, and mouth are like open doors for germs. Research has clocked us touching our faces around 23 times an hour, often near these entry points (Ref 19)! Clean hands slam that door shut, stopping germs from completing their journey into our bodies (Ref 19).

The beauty of handwashing isn't just theoretical; its impact echoes through history and across communities. Remember Ignaz Semmelweis, the 19th-century doctor who drastically reduced deaths in maternity wards simply by getting doctors to wash their hands? His discovery was revolutionary then and remains fundamental now. Modern studies consistently show that promoting handwashing in communities can slash rates of illnesses like diarrhea by nearly a third. In schools, simple hand hygiene programs mean fewer sick days, with reductions in respiratory and tummy bugs often between 20% and 50%!

You see its power everywhere when you look:

Healing Havens: Hospitals champion hand hygiene ("Clean Hands Save Lives!") as a core strategy against infections acquired during treatment. Better hand cleaning by staff leads to dramatic drops in dangerous bugs like MRSA.

Little Hands, Big Lessons: Schools and daycares teach scheduled handwashing (before snacks, after potty breaks) turning it into a healthy habit that keeps common bugs at bay, meaning more learning and less time feeling poorly.

Crisis Control: During health emergencies like the COVID-19 pandemic, handwashing became a global mantra, a simple, universal action empowering communities to slow the spread alongside other measures.

Taste of Safety: In kitchens everywhere, rigorous handwashing isn't just good practice; it's essential (and often legally required) to prevent foodborne illnesses passed from hands to food.

In the end, it might feel mundane, almost too simple to be a superpower. But the evidence is overwhelming. Cleaning our hands is one of the most effective, accessible, and affordable ways we have to protect ourselves and the people around us. It's a small act, performed by our own two hands, that creates ripples of health and well-being throughout our communities. It's quiet power, right at our fingertips.

The Unseen Shower: Why Your Cough Isn't Just Your Cough

Ever felt that tickle build, that unstoppable urge that explodes into a cough or a sneeze? It feels intensely personal, a momentary glitch in our own system. But in that instant, we become unintentional broadcasters. Imagine tiny, invisible messengers – droplets carrying whatever microscopic hitchhikers our bodies are hosting – launched into the air like microscopic confetti at a party no one wanted. They can travel surprisingly fast and far, little invisible sparks carrying the potential to ignite illness in others.

This isn't about shaming a sneeze; it's about understanding the quiet power we hold to protect the breathing space we all share. Thinking about "respiratory etiquette" isn't about rigid rules – it's about mindful gestures, small acts of kindness woven into the fabric of living together.

Catching the Sparks: The Art of the Mindful Cover-Up

So, that sneeze is coming. What's the move? Think of it like catching sparks before they land on dry tinder. A tissue is your best friend here – a soft net capturing those airborne messengers. But the story doesn't end there. That used tissue? It's now a captured sparkler. Handle it like one – straight into a lined bin it goes, sealing the deal. No tissue in sight? Time for the "Dracula move" – cough or sneeze into the crook of your elbow. Why? Your elbow doesn't shake hands, open doors, or type emails nearly as much as your hands do. It's a clever detour, keeping those potential germs off the high-traffic routes. And always, always, follow up with the unsung hero: handwashing. Whether you caught the spray in a tissue, your elbow, or thin air, washing those hands is like wiping the slate clean.

The Quiet Retreat: When Staying Home is an Act of Love

Feeling rough? That cough, the fever, the general "ugh"? The single most powerful act of community care you can perform is often the quietest: staying home. It feels counterintuitive sometimes, like we're letting people down by not showing up. But picture it differently: you're pulling up the drawbridge, temporarily halting the potential spread from your doorstep outwards. You're hitting pause on becoming an unwilling link in a chain reaction that could reach colleagues, classmates, or vulnerable people in your community. Think of it not as absence, but as a protective presence through absence. Every time someone chooses rest over pushing through illness, they're performing a quiet act of heroism, disrupting the invisible pathways of infection.

The Gentle Shield: Wearing a Mask When You Can't Stay Put

Sometimes, staying home isn't an option. Maybe you need care, or you live with others. If you're symptomatic and need to be around people, think of a simple mask as a personal filter – not necessarily filtering what comes in, but more importantly, muffling what goes out. It's like putting a soft screen over that burst of droplets from your cough or sneeze, catching a significant portion before they can embark on their journey. It's less about building a fortress for yourself and more about putting up a gentle barrier for others, a tangible sign that you're doing your part to contain the source.

Weaving the Safety Net, Together

Covering a cough, binning the tissue, washing hands, staying home when ill, masking up when necessary – these aren't just random tips. They are threads, each one vital, that we weave together to create a stronger, healthier community fabric. Each conscious action, however small it feels, is a contribution. It's the understanding that our breath, our health, and our responsibility don't end at our own skin. It's about recognizing the unseen connections between us and choosing, in those small, everyday moments, to act with care. It's the quiet superpower we all possess: the power to protect each other, one mindful breath, cough, or sneeze at a time.

The Ghost in the Room: How HMPV Plays Hide-and-Seek on Your Stuff

We all know that feeling – someone coughs nearby, and you instinctively hold your breath or turn away. We picture viruses like HMPV as tiny projectiles flying through the air. And sure, that happens. But HMPV is also a master of stealth, a microscopic stowaway clinging to the world around us long after the cough has faded.

Imagine this: someone fighting off HMPV absentmindedly touches a light switch. Hours later, you flip that same switch. Then, maybe you rub an itchy eye. Just like that, without ever sharing the same air, the virus might have found a new home. This isn't science fiction; it's the everyday reality of "fomites" – the scientific term for any object that can carry infectious germs. HMPV, like its sneaky viral cousins (think RSV), can survive for hours, sometimes even longer depending on the spot it landed on, patiently waiting on countertops, doorknobs, even clothes. These everyday items become unwitting accomplices, invisible bridges carrying the virus from one person to the next.

Shining a Light: Banishing the Viral Squatters

Knowing these invisible invaders can camp out on surfaces makes the simple act of cleaning feel like a powerful act of defense. It's about reclaiming our space. Think about the journey your hands take every single day – the remote control, your phone (let's be honest, it's practically glued to us!), the tap handle, your keyboard, the kids' favourite (and likely slobbery) toy. These aren't just objects; they're high-traffic intersections for germs. In places buzzing with people – our homes, bustling daycares, schools, offices, and hospitals – these intersections become germ superhighways.

Wiping down surfaces with soap and water is like clearing away the tumbleweeds – it helps. But to really evict viruses like HMPV, you need the disinfecting cavalry. Think of disinfectants as your secret weapon against these invisible threats. Thankfully, HMPV isn't invincible. Common household heroes like diluted bleach (used safely, of course!), alcohol-based sprays (aim for 60-70% alcohol or more), hydrogen peroxide solutions, and those handy disinfectant wipes can effectively neutralize the virus. The trick isn't just what you use, but how often. Making regular disinfecting of those "hotspot" surfaces a routine, especially in shared spaces, is like putting up roadblocks on those germ superhighways. Think of schools stepping up their cleaning game during flu season – it's the same principle, applied wisely to protect everyone.

Your Personal Space Patrol: Keeping Your Bubble Safe

Beyond the shared battlegrounds of doorknobs and counters, our personal belongings can become accidental carriers too, especially things that get up close and personal with our mouths and noses. That half-finished glass of water, the towel you just used, your toothbrush, even your lip balm or the phone you hold to your cheek – these can all become temporary homes for HMPV if you're infected.

Sharing might be caring in many situations, but when respiratory viruses are making the rounds, it's like sending a handwritten invitation to the germs. Public health folks constantly remind us: avoid sharing cups, utensils, towels, and other personal items. It's basic hygiene, but it's fundamental in stopping the spread. Picture a family where one person's feeling under the weather. Giving them their own designated cup, towel, and utensils, and being extra vigilant about wiping down the bathroom sink, can feel like simple steps, but they dramatically lower the odds of the virus spreading through the household. In dorm rooms or shared apartments, resisting the urge to take a sip from a friend's drink might feel small, but it's a smart move for everyone's health.

The Takeaway: It Takes Two (Hands and Surfaces!)

Fighting off viruses like HMPV isn't just about washing our hands (though that's incredibly important!). It's also about being mindful of the world our hands touch. HMPV's ability to linger means we need to be diligent guardians of our environment. Consistent, thoughtful cleaning and disinfection of the things we touch most often, combined with the simple wisdom of keeping personal items personal, are our best strategies. It's a two-pronged approach – protecting ourselves and protecting the spaces we share, creating a healthier environment one wipe, one wash, and one un-shared cup at a time.

Weaving Our Safety Net: Why Giving Each Other Space Matters with HMPV

Think of Human Metapneumovirus (HMPV) like an invisible cloud of glitter – when someone carrying it coughs, sneezes, or even just talks enthusiastically, tiny, potentially germ-filled droplets spray out. Sparkly, but unwanted! These droplets can float directly into someone else's airway (uh oh!) or land on things we touch, waiting for a ride to our eyes, nose, or mouth.

So, how do we politely decline this glitter shower? It boils down to being mindful of our shared space and interactions. It's not about being unfriendly; it's about being smart and caring for ourselves and the people around us.

1. The Gentle Sidestep: Steering Clear of the Sneeze Zone

You know the signs – the coughs, the sniffles, the general "under the weather" vibe. Our first instinct might be a handshake, a hug, or a pat on the back. But when respiratory bugs like HMPV are making the rounds, pulling back is the kind gesture (Ref 8).

Why it feels right (and is right): Imagine someone just sneezed – the air immediately around them is like the splash zone at a water park, but with invisible virus particles instead of water. Keeping your hands to yourself avoids picking up those particles directly. And since we all unconsciously touch our faces a lot, keeping hands germ-free breaks a major pathway for the virus to get inside. Think of it as respecting their need to recover and protecting your own health simultaneously. It's a silent act of community care. Studies on how viruses travel confirm that this close-range interaction is prime time for transmission – stepping back literally takes you out of the line of fire.

2. Creating Breathing Room: Navigating Crowds with Care

Beyond the obviously unwell, think about those times we're packed together indoors – busy waiting rooms, crowded trains, bustling cafes, especially during the late winter/early spring peak season for HMPV (Ref 25).

Why it feels right (and is right): In enclosed spaces, especially those without great airflow, those invisible droplets (and even tinier airborne bits) can linger like perfume after someone leaves a room. Giving yourself and others a bit more physical space – think an invisible hula hoop around you – lowers the chances you'll breathe in what someone else just breathed out. This isn't about suspicion; it's about dilution! More space means less concentrated virus in the air you inhale. This simple act becomes incredibly important when we think about protecting the most vulnerable among us: babies whose immune systems are still learning, beloved elders, and anyone with underlying health conditions like asthma. For them, catching HMPV can be much more serious (Ref 25 highlights this risk). Keeping a bit of distance in crowded spots is like adding an extra layer to their safety blanket. Research confirms that even a few feet can make a big difference in reducing exposure, especially over time.

Seeing it in Action: Little Bubbles of Safety Everywhere

This isn't just theory; it's woven into the fabric of how we care for each other:

Healing Havens: Hospitals space out waiting room chairs or create separate flows for potentially infectious patients

– they're building pockets of safety based on real-time virus tracking.

Little Learners: Daycares might spread out nap mats or encourage "air fives" during peak sniffle season. It's about letting kids be kids while minimizing easy germ-swapping. Fewer shared germs mean fewer missed days and healthier little bodies.

Golden Years Guardians: Nursing homes often manage visiting schedules or ensure residents aren't clustered too closely in dining areas. It's a testament to protecting those who've lived long lives, understanding that HMPV can hit them hard.

Our Daily Dance: Even offices suggesting flexible work for vulnerable employees during outbreaks, or venues improving air circulation, are embracing this principle of respectful space.

The Takeaway:

Avoiding close contact and maintaining distance aren't cold or isolating actions. They are warm, mindful strategies rooted in understanding how tiny things travel. They empower us to protect ourselves and, crucially, to shield the most vulnerable members of our community. It's about navigating our shared world with awareness and kindness, creating a healthier space for everyone, one thoughtful step back at a time.

Protecting the Vulnerable: Infection Prevention and Control in High-Risk Settings

Beyond the Headlines: Keeping Our Healthcare Spaces Safe from HMPV

You know the big names – Influenza, RSV. They get all the press. But lurking slightly out of the spotlight is Human Metapneumovirus (HMPV), a respiratory bug that can pack a serious punch, especially for the little ones, our cherished elders, and anyone whose immune system is already working overtime. Keeping this virus from spreading like wildfire in hospitals and clinics isn't just policy; it's about protecting the people we care for and the dedicated folks providing that care.

Think of our strategy like a two-layered shield: a fundamental defense we use every single day for everyone, boosted by special tactics when we know HMPV might be knocking at the door.

Layer 1: The Everyday Armor – Standard Precautions (Because Germs Don't Announce Themselves!)

This isn't about HMPV specifically; it's the baseline 'safety-first' thinking for all patient care. Why? Because we have to assume any interaction could involve invisible germs. It's about weaving safety into the very fabric of healing.

Hand Hygiene: The Undisputed Champion! Seriously, clean hands are our superpower. Washing thoroughly with soap and water or using that trusty alcohol-based rub is like kryptonite to viruses like HMPV that love to hitch rides on our hands and surfaces. It sounds simple, but study after study shows this single act dramatically cuts down infections in healthcare settings [Think: Pittet D, et al. Lancet. 2000]. It's a small action with heroic results.

Smart Protection (PPE): This isn't about dressing up like a spaceman for every task. It's about using your smarts: Might I encounter splashes? Am I getting close to someone coughing? Then grab the right gear – gloves, maybe a gown, a mask, or eye protection [Ref 14]. It's tailored protection, not just ticking a box.

Needle Safety Smarts: Keeping injections clean and sterile is non-negotiable. One needle, one syringe, one time – protecting everyone from infections spread through the bloodstream.

Clean Spaces, Healthy Places: HMPV can hang out on bed rails, doorknobs, and equipment. Regular, thorough cleaning and disinfecting isn't just tidying up; it's actively kicking germs out [Ref 14, Carling PC, et al. Clin Infect Dis. 2008]. We're scrubbing away their hiding spots!

Layer 2: Calling in the Specialists – Transmission-Based Precautions (When HMPV is the Suspect)

Okay, now we think (or know!) HMPV is in the building. Our everyday armor is still on, but we add extra defenses because this virus spreads mainly through coughs, sneezes (those pesky droplets!), and touching contaminated surfaces [Ref 14]. We deploy Droplet and Contact Precautions.

Giving HMPV Less Room to Roam (Patient Placement): Ideally, someone with HMPV gets their own room [Ref 14]. Think of it as giving the virus fewer neighbors to visit. If single rooms are scarce, we group patients with the same bug together (cohorting). It's about containing the spread and creating safe zones [See: CDC Guideline for Isolation Precautions, 2007].

Gearing Up (Dedicated PPE): Entering the room of someone with HMPV? It's time for the specific gear: a gown and gloves because the virus can be on surfaces or the patient (Contact), plus a facemask and eye protection (goggles/face shield) because of those airborne droplets [Ref 14]. We're blocking all the virus's potential entry points – hands, clothes, eyes, nose, and mouth.

Keeping Germs Contained (Limiting Transport): We try to keep patients with HMPV comfortably in their room. If they must travel through the facility (like for a necessary scan), they wear a mask, and we take special care during the journey to prevent spreading germs along the way [Ref 14].

Knowing Your Enemy: Why Testing is King

How do we know when to bring out the special tactics? Testing! Quickly finding out if someone's cough and sniffles are HMPV helps us use these extra precautions effectively – putting them in place swiftly when needed and stopping them when the coast is clear [Ref 26]. This protects everyone and helps us use our resources (like single rooms and extra PPE) wisely. Thankfully, modern tests can often spot HMPV and other culprits fast, letting us make smarter decisions sooner.

Picture This: HMPV in Action (and How We Respond)

Scenario 1: The Kids' Ward. Uh oh. Several children start coughing. Quick tests reveal HMPV. Action stations! Confirmed cases get the Droplet/Contact precautions, maybe share a designated area. Staff double down on handwashing and cleaning. New kids are watched closely for symptoms. This targeted blitz stops the outbreak in its tracks.

Scenario 2: The Care Home. An elderly resident feels unwell, showing respiratory signs. In a place where residents are more vulnerable, staff don't wait. They start Droplet and Contact precautions right away while testing is done. If HMPV is confirmed, they might check who else was exposed, step up cleaning in common areas, and perhaps adjust visiting rules for a bit to shield everyone. It's proactive protection for a precious community.

The Bottom Line

Tackling HMPV in healthcare isn't about one magic bullet. It's about a smart, layered defense. Our everyday Standard Precautions are the foundation, always there. When HMPV shows up, we add the targeted shield of Droplet and Contact Precautions, guided by sharp testing. It's vigilance, teamwork, and using every tool we have – from hand sanitizer to high-tech tests – to keep our patients safe and our healthcare heroes protected. It's how we keep everyone breathing a little easier.

Holding the Line: Protecting Our Most Vulnerable in Their Homes

Imagine walking into a place that's more than just a building; it's a home, a sanctuary for people in the later chapters of their lives. These are our parents, grandparents, cherished neighbors – individuals who carry decades of stories and wisdom, but whose bodies often bear the marks of time, making them uniquely susceptible. Long-term care homes are meant to be safe harbors, yet they stand on the front lines when invisible threats like viruses emerge. Here, an outbreak isn't just a news headline; it's a potential wildfire threatening people we deeply care about, individuals for whom even a common illness can have devastating consequences. The sad truth, shown time and again during health crises, is that these homes can suffer disproportionate losses, making our defense strategies absolutely critical – a sacred trust.

The First Whisper: Tuning into Subtle Signals

Success hinges on catching the very first spark before it can ignite. This requires more than just following procedures; it demands watchful eyes and attuned hearts from the caregivers. Recognizing that a resident seems a little quieter, slightly warmer, or just off could be the crucial first clue. It's about maintaining a gentle, constant vigilance. Quick checks, whether simple rapid tests providing immediate insights or more definitive lab tests, become essential tools – not just diagnostics, but lifelines thrown out early to identify who needs help and protection before the threat spreads widely. Think of it as hearing the faintest tremor before the earthquake; the sooner we know, the quicker we can brace for impact and limit the harm.

Sounding the Alarm: A Swift, Coordinated Embrace of Safety

Once that first signal is confirmed, there's no time for hesitation. A well-rehearsed plan must spring into action, a symphony of coordinated measures designed to shield everyone.

Protective Gear as Armor: Suddenly, masks, gowns, and gloves transform from routine supplies into essential armor. Staff don this gear meticulously, creating a physical barrier between the invisible danger and both the residents and themselves. It's a visible sign of commitment to keeping everyone safe.

Creating Safe Zones: The concept of "cohorting" becomes vital. It's about gently grouping residents – keeping those who are ill together and separate from those who might have been exposed, and importantly, from those who are still healthy. This often means dedicated teams of caregivers stay within specific zones, like loyal guards protecting their assigned areas, preventing the unintentional carrying of germs across thresholds. Real-world experience has shown this careful separation significantly slows the spread within the home's walls.

A Necessary Quiet: The lively hum of group lunches or bingo games may need to fall silent temporarily. While restricting movement and pausing communal activities is socially difficult, it's a powerful act of love – reducing the chances for the infection to hop from person to person through close contact. Studies of past outbreaks, like influenza, confirm that hitting pause quickly helps quell the spread faster.

Sanctuary Scrub: The very environment – handrails, doorknobs, shared equipment – needs extra care. Enhanced cleaning isn't just tidying up; it's actively battling the unseen enemy that can linger on surfaces. Using the right disinfectants with focused effort becomes a non-negotiable layer of defense.

Guarding the Guardians: The dedicated staff are the heart of the home, but they can also unknowingly carry threats in or out. Checking staff for symptoms before their shift, taking temperatures, and having clear rules for staying home when sick or exposed are paramount. Encouraging and facilitating vaccinations and boosters adds another strong layer to their protective shield, safeguarding both them and the residents they serve.

The Power of Shared Understanding: None of this works in a vacuum. Clear, honest, and frequent communication is the thread that ties it all together. Keeping staff updated, informing residents and their families about what's happening and why, and working hand-in-hand with public health experts builds trust and ensures everyone is moving in the same direction. When families understand the measures being taken, even the difficult ones, anxiety lessens, and cooperation strengthens.

More Than Rules: A Commitment of Heart and Science

Containing outbreaks in these special homes is a dynamic dance between vigilance, science, and deep compassion. It acknowledges the fragility of the residents and the communal nature of their home. It demands strict adherence not just to rules, but to the reasons behind them – protecting precious lives. Success lies in recognizing the heightened risk instantly and responding with a coordinated, multi-layered plan that is deployed with both precision and heart the very moment danger is suspected. It's not just infection control; it's about fiercely protecting a community.

Keeping Our Little Explorers Healthy: Making Schools & Daycares Safe Harbors

Imagine our schools and childcare centers – they're buzzing hives of discovery, laughter, and scraped knees. They're where friendships blossom and futures begin. They are, quite simply, magical places essential to our kids and our communities. But like any bustling port, these wonderful hubs can sometimes become places where unwanted visitors – like colds, flu bugs, and other pesky germs – decide to spread like wildfire.

Nobody wants learning adventures derailed by sniffles and fevers! That's why weaving simple, smart habits into the daily rhythm isn't just a good idea; it's like giving our kids, teachers, and staff invisible shields. It's about creating a culture of care, layer by layer, so everyone stays healthy and happy.

Our Toolkit for Sparkling Health:

The Power of Suds & Squirts (Hand Hygiene): Think of handwashing as a mini superpower! Twenty seconds of bubbly soap and water (sing "Happy Birthday" twice!) washes away those tiny troublemakers. Can't get to a sink? A squirt of hand sanitizer is the next best thing. It's amazing how this simple act, done often, sends so many germs packing, keeping tummy aches and coughs at bay. It's like giving germs the slip!

Catch That Cough! (Respiratory Etiquette): Achoo! A cough or sneeze can launch germs like tiny rockets. Let's teach our little ones (and remind ourselves!) the superhero move: catch that cough or sneeze in a tissue or the crook of an elbow. It's like putting up a quick deflector shield, stopping those droplets right in their tracks and protecting friends nearby.

Sparkle & Shine Patrol (Cleaning): Germs can be surprisingly clingy, hanging out on doorknobs, desks, crayons, and especially those tempting toys that toddlers love to taste-test! Making sure these high-traffic spots and shared items get regular wipe-downs disrupts the germs' travel plans. Think of it as resetting the space daily, making it gleam with health and readiness for play and learning.

The "Rest Up at Home" Rule (Stay Home When Sick): This one is huge, even if it's tricky sometimes. If a child or staff member feels unwell (think fever, cough, tummy troubles), the bravest and kindest thing they can do is stay home and rest. It's like hitting the pause button on germ-sharing. Sending a sick child to school is like sending a pirate with a cold onto a crowded ship – it rarely ends well for the crew! Clear communication between schools and families about when to stay home is key to protecting everyone.

Let the Fresh Air In! (Ventilation): Imagine clearing out a stuffy room – ahh, refreshing! Good airflow does the same for classrooms. Opening windows (when possible), making sure air systems are working well to bring in outside air, or even using air purifiers helps dilute and whisk away airborne germs that might be floating around. Think of it as giving the air itself a good spring clean, making it harder for germs to linger. Sometimes, checking CO2 levels can even give us clues about how fresh the air really is!

Stronger Together: The Layering Magic

None of these steps is a magic bullet on its own. The real power comes when we layer them together. Consistent handwashing plus catching coughs plus clean surfaces plus staying home when sick plus fresh air... that's our winning combination! It creates overlapping shields of protection.

When we embrace these practices, we're not just fighting germs; we're actively building healthier, more resilient spaces for our youngest learners to thrive. We're minimizing sick days, keeping the learning buzz going strong, and protecting not just the kids and staff in the building, but their families and communities too. Let's make these simple acts of care part of the everyday magic in our schools and childcare centers!

Building a Sanctuary: Cocooning Those Who Walk a Fragile Path

Imagine living in a world where a common cold isn't just an inconvenience, but a potential catastrophe. For some incredible people navigating life – perhaps bravely facing cancer, cherishing the gift of a transplanted organ, managing advanced HIV, or born with an immune system that simply doesn't have the usual defenses – this is their reality. Their bodies, already working so hard, face an overwhelming battle against everyday germs [Evidence: We see this starkly in medical studies showing how infections like the flu, COVID-19, or RSV can have devastating consequences for them compared to others; journals like The Lancet frequently document this heightened risk]. Even our modern miracles, like vaccines, often don't offer them the same sturdy shield they give the rest of us; their immune response can be like a whisper instead of a shout [Fact: Think of COVID-19 vaccines – while highly effective for most, studies from places like Johns Hopkins showed that sometimes fewer than half of transplant recipients developed strong protection, compared to over 90% in healthy folks].

This reality calls for more than just standard advice; it requires us to consciously build a sanctuary, layer by protective layer, around them.

Guardians at the Gate: Protection Begins at Home and in Our Communities

The first threads of this safety net are woven right into daily life. It starts with open, honest conversations with patients and their families. Yes, washing hands frequently is crucial – almost a ritual of care. But it also means being mindful of the invisible threats lingering on doorknobs, phones, and counters, making regular disinfection a quiet act of defense [Evidence: Science shows us viruses can survive on surfaces for hours or even days, waiting for a chance].

Crowded places, especially stuffy indoor ones, become landscapes to navigate with extreme caution, regardless of the season [Evidence: We know respiratory viruses love to travel through the air in packed spaces, a risk magnified for those whose bodies can't easily fight back]. And perhaps one of the hardest parts: needing to gently steer clear of anyone, even loved ones, who feels even slightly unwell. That minor sniffle for you could mean a serious lung infection for them [Evidence: Sadly, studies often show that infections in vulnerable individuals trace back to close, everyday contacts].

Masking also takes on a deeper meaning. Forget debates about mandates; for someone profoundly immunocompromised, and for those who share their immediate space, a high-quality mask (like an N95 or KN95) worn consistently in public indoor settings becomes a personal shield, a portable clean-air bubble [Evidence: Research, including thorough reviews by groups like Cochrane, confirms that good masks, especially respirators, genuinely reduce the chance of spreading or catching respiratory bugs]. It's not about living in fear; it's about making informed, loving choices to minimize risk.

Within Healing Walls: Fortifying Healthcare Havens

Inside hospitals and clinics, where vulnerable people gather and germs can concentrate, the need for vigilance skyrockets. For those most at risk, like bone marrow transplant recipients, special "protective environments" become essential. These aren't just rooms; they're safe zones with air meticulously filtered (using HEPA systems) and pressurized to keep out dangerous invaders like airborne fungal spores [Evidence: Hospitals have seen dramatic drops, sometimes over 50%, in dangerous fungal infections after installing these air filtration systems in sensitive units].

The commitment extends to every single person entering their space. Staff and visitors don protective gear – often top-tier masks, gowns, gloves – not just for specific procedures, but routinely, creating layers of defense [Evidence: Infection control guidelines from organizations like the CDC stress this, as breaches in protocol are known causes of outbreaks]. Visitors might face careful screening questions about symptoms or recent exposures, and visiting times might be limited, all to protect a fragile peace [Fact: Hospitals routinely enact stricter visiting rules for these units, especially when viruses are circulating widely in the community].

Looking Ahead: Arming the Vulnerable with Future Shields

Thinking proactively is paramount. While vaccines might not provide complete armor, every bit helps, so optimizing schedules and extra doses are still important. For a time, lab-created antibodies (like Evusheld against COVID-19) offered a crucial shield for those who couldn't make their own, though we learned these shields need constant updating as viruses cleverly change shape [Evidence: Early studies showed these antibodies worked well, but later research confirmed they lost effectiveness against newer virus variants, showing the ongoing need for innovation]. The hope now rests on the next wave of defenses – perhaps powerful antiviral pills taken preventatively or new antibodies designed to outsmart a wider range of viral tricks. When these arrive, you can be sure these vulnerable groups will be first in line.

Bringing it to Life: Stories of Sanctuary in Action

The Transplant Floor: Picture a hospital's transplant unit during a winter surge of RSV. They don't just wait and see. They immediately require top-grade masks for everyone on the floor, meticulously screen visitors, keep potentially ill patients separate, and actively remind every transplant patient about staying safe outside the hospital – maybe suggesting home air purifiers or skipping large family gatherings. It's a proactive defense against an invisible siege.

The Children's Cancer Clinic: Imagine a cheerful-looking clinic for kids fighting leukemia. Behind the scenes, a "low-risk pathway" is carefully managed. Families might be advised to create a protective "bubble" at home, maybe having siblings mask up at school during flu season. In the clinic, HEPA filters hum quietly in waiting areas, playtime is managed to avoid too much close contact, and staff are extra vigilant with masks and gloves. The result? Fewer scary fevers and emergency visits caused by common viruses, a testament to these layers of care.

Ultimately, shielding those with the most fragile immune systems isn't a checklist; it's a living commitment. It's a dynamic dance between doctors, nurses, patients, families, and the wider community, constantly adapting to the person's needs, the germs currently circulating, and the best tools science can offer. It's weaving a strong, flexible, and deeply human safety net, together.

The Quest for an HMPV Vaccine: Progress, Platforms, and Persistent Challenges (2025)

The Unseen Heavyweight in the Ring: Why We Need to Take HMPV Seriously

Think about the viruses that make headlines every winter. Influenza struts in, bold and notorious. RSV often follows, infamous for filling pediatric wards. We know their names, we brace for their arrival. But there's another contender in the ring, a quieter, often overlooked heavyweight that lands significant blows: Human Metapneumovirus, or HMPV.

Since scientists finally put a name to its face back in 2001, we've realized HMPV isn't some newcomer. It's been among us for ages, a shadow player contributing significantly to the coughs, fevers, and respiratory distress that sweep through our communities year after year. It's not just another cold virus; it's a major reason why so many hospital beds fill up, why parents spend sleepless nights listening to their child's wheezing, and why vulnerable people face serious health threats.

More Than Just a "Bad Cold": The Real Toll of HMPV

Imagine a bustling children's hospital during peak season. Tiny chests struggling for breath, the beep of monitors, worried parents pacing hallways. While RSV often gets the spotlight, HMPV is right there beside it, responsible for a big chunk – sometimes up to 15% – of those scary respiratory illnesses that land kids in the hospital. It looks a lot like RSV – bronchiolitis, pneumonia – but it packs its own unique punch, adding dramatically to the strain on our healthcare heroes and resources. It's the reason why "just a virus" can turn into days or weeks of intensive care for the smallest among us.

And it's not just about the little ones. Think about our grandparents, residents in nursing homes, or anyone whose immune system is already working overtime fighting other battles – like cancer patients or transplant recipients. For them, catching HMPV isn't a minor inconvenience. It can be a devastating blow, leading to severe pneumonia, worsening existing lung conditions, prolonged hospital stays, and tragically, sometimes stealing precious time. Picture an outbreak stealthily spreading through a care facility – it's a scenario that plays out too often, highlighting a critical vulnerability.

The Ripple Effect: Costs Beyond Hospital Walls

The impact doesn't stop at the bedside. Every HMPV hospitalization rings up costs – for intensive care, tests, treatments. But the economic drain flows further: parents missing critical workdays to care for sick children, adults sidelined from their jobs, productivity dipping across businesses. It's a silent drain on families' finances and the broader economy, a cost we collectively bear, often without even naming the culprit.

Fighting Blindfolded? The Treatment Gap

Here's a crucial part of the story: we're fighting this significant threat with limited tools. Unlike the flu, where we have specific antiviral medications, there's no targeted weapon against HMPV. Doctors and nurses provide incredible supportive care – oxygen, fluids, fever control – but they lack a specific tool to stop the virus itself.

Yes, washing hands, covering coughs, staying home when sick – these are absolutely vital first lines of defense. They help slow the spread of all respiratory bugs. But let's be honest, they aren't enough to stop HMPV in its tracks, especially when it spreads so easily through schools, homes, and healthcare settings. It's like trying to hold back a flood with sandbags when what you really need is a dam.

The Call to Action: Forging the Missing Shield

This is where the story needs to change. Faced with a virus that causes widespread illness, hits our most vulnerable the hardest, costs us dearly, and lacks specific treatments, the path forward becomes clear. A vaccine isn't just a "nice-to-have"; it's the missing shield in our public health armory.

Imagine a future where fewer children gasp for breath in emergency rooms because of HMPV. Where elderly loved ones are better protected from severe pneumonia. Where immunocompromised individuals have one less threat to fear. Where healthcare systems can breathe a little easier during respiratory season.

Developing an HMPV vaccine is about more than preventing illness; it's about investing in healthier childhoods, safer aging, reduced healthcare burdens, and stronger communities. It's time to bring HMPV out of the shadows and meet this challenge head-on. It's time to build that shield.

The Unseen Threat and the Race Against Time: Chasing the HMPV Vaccine in 2025

Imagine a virus, a stealthy cousin to the notorious RSV, that slips under the radar for most, causing sniffles and coughs. But for tiny babies battling for breath in hospital cribs, or for grandparents suddenly facing serious pneumonia, Human Metapneumovirus (HMPV) is anything but minor. It's a significant health burden, packing a punch nearly as hard as RSV in some hospital wards, yet it's remained a frustratingly elusive target for vaccine developers since its discovery back in 2001.

But the tide is turning. As 2025 unfolds, the quest for an HMPV vaccine isn't just simmering; it's boiling over. Fueled by hard-won lessons from the recent RSV vaccine breakthroughs and a growing recognition of HMPV's impact, labs and biotech firms are locked in a high-stakes race, armed with cutting-edge science and innovative strategies.

The 'Secret Weapon': Locking Onto the Shapeshifting Protein

The breakthrough moment? Realizing the virus's own "key" – its fusion (F) protein – was the target. But not just any version of it. Scientists learned from RSV that they needed to catch this protein before it shapeshifts to unlock our cells. This delicate "prefusion" form is the holy grail. It's like learning to disarm a bomb before it's primed. Now, the challenge is to create vaccines that showcase this specific, vulnerable shape to our immune system. Teams like those at Scripps Research are like molecular sculptors, carefully tweaking the protein's structure to make it more stable, crafting the perfect training dummy for our body's defenses.

An Arsenal of Innovation: Diverse Strategies Converge

The approaches are as diverse as they are ingenious:

mRNA Magic: Fresh off its world-changing success with COVID-19, mRNA technology is being repurposed. Think of

Moderna's candidate (mRNA-1653) – not just aiming at HMPV, but also tackling another respiratory troublemaker, PIV3, in one shot. Early peeks show it's well-tolerated and successfully rallies antibody troops in both toddlers and adults, urging development forward.

Clever Decoys (VLPs): Imagine building a perfect replica of the enemy tank, but without the engine or guns. That's the idea behind Virus-Like Particles (VLPs). AstraZeneca, having teamed up with Icosavax, is pushing IVX-A12 – a VLP armed with those crucial prefusion F proteins from both RSV and HMPV. It's already aced early safety and immune-boosting tests in older adults and was declared "Phase 3 ready" as 2024 dawned. Now deep into further trials, it's a major contender. Others, like Clover Biopharmaceuticals, are hot on their heels, prepping their own protein-based candidates for 2025 trials.

Taming the Beast (LAVs): Some are betting on using a weakened, "live but attenuated" version of HMPV itself to teach the immune system. Metavac®-RSV, for example, is designed as a nasal spray hoping to offer dual protection against HMPV and RSV, showing promise in early animal studies.

Trojan Horses (Vector Vaccines): Another tactic involves using a harmless virus as a delivery truck, sneaking in the HMPV blueprints (antigens) to trigger immunity.

Stronger Together: The Power of Combination

A striking theme? Hitting two (or even three) birds with one stone. Since HMPV and RSV often circulate together, attacking the same vulnerable groups, combination vaccines just make sense. Simplify vaccine schedules, broaden protection – it's a win-win. Beyond AstraZeneca's dual-action shot, Vicebio is making waves with VXB-241 (RSV/HMPV), powered by unique "Molecular Clamp" tech and backed by hefty funding. They're expecting initial results mid-2025 and are already planning a triple-threat vaccine (VXB-251) adding PIV3. And don't forget the "Rhyme" study, where giants University of Oxford and Moderna are testing an mRNA combo specifically in infants, aiming to shield the tiniest patients from the very start.

Where Science Meets Humanity: The Real-World Test

These aren't just lab experiments. The ongoing trials are where the rubber meets the road. IVX-A12 is being tested in the very grandparents HMPV often hospitalizes. The Rhyme study directly targets the frightening vulnerability of infants. Success here means translating complex science into tangible relief: fewer emergency room visits, less strain on hospitals, and families breathing easier. Scientists are even developing controlled "human challenge" models – safely exposing volunteers – to potentially speed up the verdict on which vaccines truly work.

While the finish line – a licensed HMPV vaccine on pharmacy shelves – hasn't been crossed yet, the air crackles with potential. The convergence of different technologies, the laser focus on that prefusion protein, and the powerful momentum behind combination vaccines paint the most optimistic picture yet. The next few years could finally see us gain the upper hand against this long-overlooked respiratory foe.

The Ghost in the Machine: Wrestling with Past Shadows

First, there's a ghost story that haunts this field. Decades ago, scientists tried to make a shield against HMPV's close cousin, RSV. But something went wrong. The early attempt, using an older method, seemed to backfire. Instead of protecting babies, it tragically made some sicker when they later met the real virus. It was like the shield accidentally painted a target on them. Because HMPV and RSV are family, researchers walk cautiously. Every new idea for an HMPV shield is tested with this "what if?" echoing in the background. They need absolute certainty that the shield won't turn into a target. Modern science, thankfully, has smarter tools now, focusing on specific parts of the virus (like its 'entry key' in a particular shape) believed to be much safer, aiming to banish that ghost for good.

The Guarded Gates: Protecting Our Littlest Ones

Think about newborns. They arrive with a temporary, hand-me-down shield borrowed from their mothers – antibodies passed along before birth. It's a beautiful gift, nature's head start. But this borrowed shield can be tricky. When scientists try to teach the baby's own immune system to build a permanent shield (with a vaccine), those helpful maternal antibodies can sometimes get in the way. They might grab onto the vaccine, like overeager guards, preventing the baby's system from learning the lesson properly. It's a delicate dance: figuring out the perfect moment to train the baby's defenses, just as the borrowed shield starts to fade, or designing a vaccine lesson that these 'guards' don't intercept.

The Weathered Immune System: Reaching Our Elders

At the other end of life's journey, our elders face a different hurdle. Their immune systems are like veteran soldiers – experienced, but perhaps a bit slower to react, a bit harder of hearing. Scientists call this 'immunosenescence.' It means that a standard vaccine 'call to arms' might not be loud enough to rally a strong defense. This is crucial because HMPV can hit seniors hard, leading to serious lung infections. So, the quest here is to create a vaccine signal that's loud and clear – maybe a stronger dose, or adding a special 'megaphone' (an adjuvant) to make sure the message gets through and the veteran defenses stand ready.

The Enemy's Disguises: A Virus That Changes Its Coat

HMPV itself isn't one single entity. It's more like a family with different members (A's and B's, with slightly different 'coats'). Sometimes Type A is common, other times Type B, and they can swap dominance year to year. A truly useful shield needs to protect against all the common family members. Researchers are focusing on parts of the virus that don't change much between strains – like that essential 'entry key' again – hoping to create a master key that unlocks protection no matter which coat the virus is wearing that season.

An Echo, Not a Shout: Immunity That Fades

Catching HMPV once doesn't mean you're safe forever. People get reinfected throughout life, although later infections are often milder. This tells us that our body's natural 'memory' of HMPV fades over time. It's likely a vaccine-induced memory will also dim. So, the shield might need polishing. Booster shots, especially for those most at risk, might be necessary to keep the protection strong. Figuring out when to polish the shield will be part of the ongoing story even after a vaccine is available.

Fitting In: The Crowded World of Childhood Shots

Finally, imagine trying to add another tool to an already packed toolbox. New childhood vaccines often need to fit into the existing shot schedule, sometimes combined with other vaccines into a single injection to make things easier for parents and kids. Creating an HMPV component that plays nicely with others – ensuring it works perfectly without weakening the effect of its companions, and vice-versa – adds another layer of careful engineering and testing.

The Modern Quest: Tools for the Task

Today's explorers are using cutting-edge maps and tools:

mRNA blueprints: Like sending precise instructions (similar to some COVID-19 vaccines) telling our cells exactly how to build a piece of the HMPV shield (often that 'entry key'). This tech is fast and potentially powerful, especially for waking up those 'veteran' immune systems in the elderly.

Tamed viruses: Using a weakened version of HMPV itself, trained to teach the immune system without causing illness. It's a delicate balance – making it gentle enough for babies but strong enough to teach effectively.

Precision pieces: Selecting just key proteins from the virus (like the 'entry key') and presenting them, often with those 'megaphones' (adjuvants), to focus the immune response, particularly valuable for older adults.

Each clinical trial is like a field expedition, gathering vital intelligence: Is it safe? Does it work well in babies and grandparents? Does it protect against the virus's different disguises? How long does the shield last? Navigating this complex landscape, haunted by past shadows, complicated by age, and challenged by a shape-shifting virus, is the human journey towards finally shielding everyone from HMPV.

Finally, Hope Takes Flight Against HMPV: A Vaccine Horizon We Can Almost Touch

For years, Human Metapneumovirus (HMPV) has been like the quieter, often-ignored sibling hovering in the shadow of its more notorious respiratory cousin, RSV. While RSV grabbed headlines, HMPV quietly continued its work, filling hospital beds and causing genuine distress, especially for the very young and the elderly. But now? A real sense of optimism is bubbling up, almost palpable, and it's being supercharged by incredible leaps in vaccine science (Ref 26).

Think about the technologies that recently gave us powerful tools against other challenging viruses – the elegant precision of mRNA, the cleverness of viral vectors, the targeted approach of subunit proteins. These aren't just tweaks; they're revolutionary blueprints. And now, these same cutting-edge platforms are being aimed squarely at HMPV (Ref 26). It feels like we're finally giving this underdog virus the attention it deserves, armed with twenty-first-century weapons.

If these efforts hit the mark and deliver a licensed vaccine, the change could be nothing short of transformative. Picture this: the terrifying rates of severe lung infections like bronchiolitis and pneumonia, driven by HMPV, begin to fall dramatically. Imagine the collective sigh of relief from parents watching their infants breathe easier, and the reduced anxiety in elder care homes during peak virus season (Ref 26). This isn't just about dodging a bad cold; it's about preventing those harrowing hospital stays, the ones marked by beeping machines and worried faces. Think of pediatric wards with more empty beds, freeing up dedicated healthcare workers. Studies have shown HMPV can account for a hefty slice (5-10%) of kids' respiratory hospital trips – imagine shrinking that number significantly! Consequently, the immense pressure HMPV puts on our entire healthcare system could ease, saving not just suffering, but resources, allowing caregivers and patients to avoid missed days of work and school (Ref 26).

Cleverly, scientists are looking at the recent triumphs in the RSV vaccine arena and seeing a strategic advantage. Why not create a dynamic duo, a bivalent vaccine that tackles both RSV and HMPV? (Ref 2, 26). It makes perfect sense. These two troublemakers often arrive together, target the same vulnerable little lungs (and older ones), and cause illnesses that doctors can barely tell apart. A combo shot could mean broader protection with fewer jabs – a win for immunization schedules and potentially making it easier for everyone to get protected. We can essentially ride the wave of innovation, knowledge, and even the regulatory pathways already smoothed out by the new RSV vaccines, potentially fast-tracking HMPV protection (Ref 2, 26). It's like learning from one successful mission to launch an even bigger, better one.

But having a brilliant vaccine candidate is just the start of the story. Turning that scientific sparkle into real-world health requires thoughtful choreography. Big questions loom: How do we smoothly integrate an HMPV vaccine (or the RSV/HMPV combo) into the already packed schedule of shots kids and adults receive? Nailing the timing and dose is key. Who needs it most urgently? Logically, it would be babies heading into their first HMPV season and perhaps older adults with higher risks, but figuring out the rollout needs careful, ethical planning. And crucially, once a vaccine is out there, we need to become tireless watchdogs. Establishing robust systems to monitor how well it really works across different communities, to catch any rare side effects, and to understand how long the protection lasts is non-negotiable. This constant listening and learning builds trust and allows us to fine-tune our approach, ensuring the shield remains strong (Ref 2, 26).

So yes, the future for HMPV vaccination looks incredibly promising, brighter than it ever has before (Ref 26). But translating that laboratory light into widespread well-being requires a full-court press: brilliant science, smart regulation, practical rollout plans, and ongoing vigilance (Ref 2, 26). The potential reward – lifting the heavy weight of HMPV from countless shoulders globally – makes this complex, challenging journey absolutely worth undertaking. We're not just forging ahead; we're forging hope.

HMPV in Practice - Case Studies Part 1: Illustrating Diverse Presentations and Diagnostics

Maya's Fight: A Whisper That Became a Roar

Four months. That's how long Maya had been gracing the world, a tiny soul who'd entered the scene a bit early, eight weeks ahead of schedule. Her first breaths hadn't been in the calm final weeks of gestation but in the bright intensity of the NICU. Her lungs, like delicate, unfinished blossoms, carried the memory of that early start [Ref 19]. Back home, she was a quiet miracle, hitting her milestones in her own sweet time, her parents charting every precious gain.

But winter arrived, not just with frosted windows, but with an invisible army of seasonal viruses, including the notorious Human Metapneumovirus (HMPV) [Ref 5]. It started softly, almost apologetically – a little cough. Easy to wave away as just a cold. But this wasn't just a cold. Within two days, the gentle cough transformed. It deepened, rattling in her tiny chest like pebbles in a jar. Breathing wasn't easy anymore; it was work. Her parents watched, hearts tightening, as the skin beneath her ribs pulled inward with each desperate gasp (retractions). A faint, high-pitched whistle (wheeze), like wind through a keyhole, joined the struggle [Ref 5, 19]. Her breaths came faster, faster (tachypnea), a frantic tempo replacing her usual peaceful rhythm. Then, the sight that sends panic through any parent: a subtle, dusky blue shadowing her lips. The unspoken signal for help, now. The emergency department beckoned.

Walking into the bright lights of the pediatric ED, Maya was the picture of bronchiolitis, holding on but clearly struggling. Her breath count was sky-high, and the pulse oximeter clipped to her tiny finger showed oxygen levels dipping into the high 80s – her little body wasn't getting enough air [Ref 19]. Through the stethoscope, the doctors heard the story her lungs were telling: a widespread chorus of wheezes and crackles, the soundtrack of inflamed lower airways [Ref 19]. Her prematurity wasn't just a fact in her history; it was a flashing red light. Babies born early, like Maya, often face a tougher battle with viruses like HMPV. Their airways are narrower, their lungs might carry lingering vulnerabilities (like bronchopulmonary dysplasia), and their immune systems are still learning the ropes [Ref 19]. It's a known, harsh reality: these tiny warriors are far more likely to need hospital care for bronchiolitis, and HMPV is often the unwelcome guest causing the havoc [Ref 5, 19].

To identify the specific virus orchestrating this chaos, a gentle swab from Maya's nose was sent for a high-tech test – a multiplex PCR panel. Think of it as a rapid identification lineup for common respiratory culprits [Ref 26]. This powerful tool is a cornerstone in modern pediatric care, pinpointing the exact virus quickly and accurately, guiding treatment, and helping track outbreaks [Ref 26]. The result came back: Human Metapneumovirus (HMPV). The suspicion was confirmed [Ref 26]. While RSV often gets the headlines, HMPV is a significant player, filling hospital beds with young children, the elderly, and those with weakened defenses, driving a considerable chunk (estimated 5-15%) of pediatric respiratory hospitalizations each year [Ref 5].

For Maya, there was no magic bullet, no specific HMPV-busting medicine. The battle plan was one of unwavering support, letting her own body fight the invader while clinicians managed the battlefield [Ref 5]. Major guidelines agree: for typical viral bronchiolitis, treatments like routine puffers (bronchodilators) or steroids often don't help and aren't recommended [Ref 5, AAP Guidelines]. The focus was pure, essential care:

Whispers of Oxygen: A thin tube beneath her nose delivered a gentle stream of oxygen, lifting those critical saturation numbers above 90-92%, easing the strain on her struggling lungs caused by the inflammation and sticky mucus [Ref 5]. Constant monitoring ensured she got just what she needed.

Clearing the Path: Tiny noses get easily blocked, and babies need to breathe through their noses. Gentle suctioning, especially before trying to feed, cleared the mucus, making each breath a little less work, a little more effective [Ref 5]. While it primarily offers comfort and clearer upper airways, it was a vital part of easing her distress.

Silent Hydration: Breathing that fast is thirsty work, and feeding becomes difficult. An IV drip initially provided the fluids she desperately needed, keeping dehydration at bay and her electrolytes balanced [Ref 5]. As the storm began to pass, she could slowly return to the comfort of feeding.

Maya's hospital room became a bubble of watchful waiting. For several days, the rhythm was set by the beep of monitors and the quiet dedication of the staff. Slowly, surely, the tide turned. Her breathing softened, the frantic pace eased. The need for extra oxygen lessened, then vanished. She started feeding with more interest, her little body signaling its recovery. Finally, the day came for discharge, her parents armed with knowledge and instructions for continued care at home [Ref 5].

Maya's Echo: Why Her Story Matters

Maya's journey, though unique to her and her family, echoes in pediatric wards everywhere, especially when viruses hold seasonal sway. Her "classic" case shines a light on real-time clinical truths:

Seeing the Risk: Knowing that prematurity drastically raises the stakes [Ref 19] helps doctors triage effectively, giving babies like Maya the closer watch they need right from the start.

Smart Testing, Not Guessing: Her symptoms pointed towards a virus, making the multiplex PCR [Ref 26] the right move, confirming HMPV, avoiding pointless antibiotics, and informing necessary isolation precautions.

Planning for the Wave: Hospitals brace for bronchiolitis season. Understanding HMPV's role [Ref 5] helps them anticipate the surge, managing beds and staff proactively.

Bridging Fear with Facts: Explaining why supportive care (oxygen, fluids) is the treatment, and what to expect, empowers parents, turning anxiety into partnership during a frightening time.

The Bigger Picture: Every confirmed HMPV case, like Maya's, adds a piece to the public health puzzle, tracking the virus's ebb and flow and fueling the quest for future defenses, like vaccines.

Maya's story is a powerful narrative of vulnerability met with resilience, highlighting the crucial dance between a baby's fighting spirit and the supportive care that helps them win against common, yet potentially serious, respiratory illnesses [Ref 5, 19]. It's a reminder of the fragility of new life and the incredible strength found in careful, compassionate medical support.

Mr. Harrison's Storm: When Familiar Walls Can't Hold Back the Tide

Imagine Mr. Harrison, 78 years etched onto his face, living within the familiar rhythm of his long-term care home. His body already carries its own history – lungs that have worked hard against the grip of COPD, a heart that beats with the careful cadence dictated by CHF (Ref 18). These aren't just diagnoses; they are constant companions, shaping his breath, his energy, his daily life.

Then, a subtle shift, like the air before a storm. His cough, usually a gruff background note, deepens, taking on a harsher, more persistent edge. A warmth spreads through him, unfamiliar and unwelcome – a fever breaking stubborn ground. The simple act of breathing, already a conscious effort, becomes a steeper climb, leaving him gasping even in the quiet stillness of his room. And perhaps most terrifying, the small device clipped to his finger begins to cry out – a digital alarm signaling that the very oxygen his body craves is slipping away (hypoxia) (Ref 18).

This isn't just a cold. This is an invasion. Severe, complicated pneumonia has breached his defenses. For residents like Mr. Harrison, the safe harbor of a care facility paradoxically becomes a place of heightened risk. Statistics tell a stark story – pneumonia strikes here ten times more often than in the wider community, and for those needing hospital care, the battle can be lost in up to half the cases, a grim reality shaped by age and underlying conditions.

Seeing Through the Fog: The Challenge of Knowing

Finding the enemy within isn't always straightforward. Mr. Harrison's daily struggles with COPD can mimic the early signs of infection, creating a dangerous camouflage. Age, too, can play tricks, sometimes silencing the typical alarms of high fever or the sharp stab of pleuritic pain. Even the trusty chest X-ray, often the first line of sight, can be like peering through fog, its images clouded by the permanent changes wrought by COPD or the fluid shifts of a struggling heart (CHF).

This is where medicine needs sharper eyes and ears. Imagine sending microscopic scouts into the battlefield – that's what Polymerase Chain Reaction (PCR) testing does. From a simple swab or sputum sample, it rapidly unmasks the specific invader, whether it's a common bacterium like Streptococcus pneumoniae or a stealthy virus like Influenza (Ref 29). Knowing the enemy's name transforms the fight, allowing doctors to choose the right weapon (antibiotic) instead of firing blindly. It's like switching from buckshot to a targeted rifle.

And for a deeper look at the battlefield itself, the Computed Tomography (CT) scan offers an unparalleled view. It slices through the shadows, revealing the extent of the damage – hidden pockets of infection (infiltrates), solidified lung tissue (consolidations), or dangerous complications like fluid collections (effusions) or abscesses that a standard X-ray might miss (Ref 29). This detailed map is crucial for gauging the severity and planning the counter-attack.

The Fight Back: A Symphony of Support

Launching a defense for Mr. Harrison is an urgent, multi-front effort, often beginning even before all the reconnaissance is complete (Ref 37):

Securing the Air Supply: Oxygen flows immediately, a vital lifeline to push back the encroaching hypoxia, aiming to restore his levels to a safer harbor (typically above 90-92%). Sometimes, more powerful support, like a breathing mask (non-invasive ventilation) or even a ventilator, is needed to win this crucial battle for breath.

The Delicate Balance of Fluids: Like tending a drought-stricken land next to a flood-prone river, managing fluids is critical. IV fluids combat dehydration from fever and rapid breathing, but too much could overwhelm his already strained heart (CHF). It requires constant vigilance – watching weight, assessing fluid status, listening to the heart's signals – a true balancing act.

The Antibiotic Assault: Time is the enemy. A powerful, broad-spectrum antibiotic combination is unleashed swiftly to fight the most likely bacterial culprits, including the tough, resistant "superbugs" sometimes found in healthcare settings (Ref 37). Think of it as an initial barrage. Once PCR or cultures identify the specific villain and its weaknesses, the attack is refined, switching to a more targeted weapon – a core principle of using these precious medicines wisely (antibiotic stewardship).

Reinforcing Existing Defenses: The pneumonia doesn't just attack the lungs; it stresses Mr. Harrison's entire system, threatening to destabilize his COPD and CHF. His care team must simultaneously fine-tune his inhalers, adjust diuretics, or modify heart medications – shoring up the ramparts of his underlying conditions is just as vital (Ref 37).

The Supporting Corps: Victory requires more than just fighting the infection. It needs good nutrition to fuel the body, gentle movement to prevent blood clots and muscle wasting, and watchful eyes for any complications – like the infection spreading (sepsis) or other organs faltering.

Beyond the Bedside: Lessons from Mr. Harrison's Struggle

Mr. Harrison's fight isn't just his own; it reflects broader challenges and inspires ongoing efforts:

Early Warning Sentinels: Can we create better systems within LTCFs to catch subtle signs of decline earlier, triggering life-saving interventions sooner?

Smarter Weapon Use: How do we best use our powerful antibiotics now, while preserving them for the future? Research into stewardship programs and rapid diagnostics in LTCFs is key.

Building Stronger Shields: Ensuring residents have their flu shots and pneumonia vaccines is like reinforcing the castle walls before the siege begins.

Bridging the Gaps: When residents move between the LTCF and hospital, clear communication and careful coordination are paramount to prevent dangerous fumbles.

Understanding True Resilience: Beyond diagnoses, how does overall frailty – that sense of vulnerability – impact recovery? Recognizing and measuring frailty helps predict risk and tailor care.

In the end, caring for Mr. Harrison is a complex tapestry woven from rapid assessment, sophisticated diagnostics like PCR and CT, and a comprehensive, human-centered response. It demands not just medical knowledge, but vigilance, empathy, and a commitment to seeing the individual navigating the storm within the disease. His vulnerability underscores the critical need for innovation and compassion in the unique world of long-term care.

The Ghost in the Throat: Why Your 'Nothing' Cold is a Secret Super-Spreader

Meet Alex. Thirty-five, healthy, life humming along. Then comes that Tuesday morning. A faint sandpaper scratch at the back of the throat. A nose that feels... aware of itself. A tiny, dry cough that punctuates the silence now and then. Annoying? Sure. A showstopper? Not even close. Deadlines are barking, the fridge is empty, life doesn't hit pause for a tickle.

Sound familiar? It's the universal shrug-off. Especially when the calendar leans towards late winter or early spring, this could easily be the quiet calling card of something like Human Metapneumovirus (HMPV) – a less-famous cousin to the flu, but a real player in the respiratory game, often dressing up as just this kind of mild annoyance in adults. It's one of the usual suspects, mingling with rhinoviruses and others, causing that "meh" feeling.

Here's the pivot: Alex, like almost everyone else feeling this way, isn't calling the doctor. Why would they? It's just a cold. No dramatic fever, no gasping for air. It's the cue for the home-remedy shuffle: more tea, maybe a lozenge, try to snag an extra hour of sleep. No swabs, no tests, no official diagnosis. The specific virus pulling the strings remains nameless, unseen. Alex's minor battle flies completely under the official health radar, a blip too small for the sophisticated surveillance systems hungry for lab reports.

But while Alex feels only slightly inconvenienced, they've unknowingly become a tiny, mobile transmitter. That little cough in the elevator? The sneeze muffled into an elbow near the coffee machine? Sharing a keyboard? Unbeknownst to Alex, the virus (HMPV, or one of its brethren) is seizing its chance, catching invisible currents to find its next host.

This is the quiet, relentless engine driving so much of what we call "cold and flu season." These millions of tiny, untested, "I'm-fine-really" infections are the massive, hidden reservoir keeping these viruses perpetually in circulation. Think of that famous iceberg: the scary hospitalizations are the gleaming tip we see and fear. But the real power, the immense, submerged bulk that keeps the whole thing afloat? That's Alex. That's millions of Alexes, soldiering on through their sniffles. It's the collective weight of countless minor infections, passed along in grocery aisles, offices, and living rooms by people who feel "well enough."

What This Secret Network Means:

The Health Detective's Dilemma: Public health folks are trying to track these bugs, but how do you count ghosts? They watch for clusters of "flu-like" symptoms, but without tests, knowing which virus is surging (Is it HMPV this week? A garden-variety coronavirus?) is like trying to map a city by only looking at the streetlights. Understanding this vast sea of mild illness is key to truly grasping a virus's impact and bracing for seasonal waves.

The Office Outbreak Origin Story: Alex showing up to work, feeling "mostly okay," is how outbreaks ignite. This "presenteeism" – pushing through minor illness – turns workplaces and schools into accidental incubators. That bug that rips through the team? It likely started with someone battling "just a cold." Maybe it's time we rethink what "toughing it out" really means when it comes to shared air.

Fueling the Future Fight: Why chase vaccines for the "common cold"? Because the combined impact isn't common; it's colossal. Pinpointing the burden of specific viruses like HMPV, including these mild cases that drive transmission to more vulnerable people (kids, the elderly, the immunocompromised), builds the case for targeted weapons – better vaccines, smarter treatments. It's not just about Alex feeling better; it's about protecting the entire network.

So, the next time you feel that familiar tickle, remember Alex. That simple, self-managed cold might feel like a personal footnote, easily ignored. But from a bigger perspective, it's a vital, humming part of the unseen machinery that keeps respiratory viruses woven into the fabric of our communities. It's the ghost in the throat that fuels the fire.

The Sound That Stops a Parent's Heart

It starts with a sound. Not a cough, not a cry, but a thin, whistling gasp that cuts through the noise of the pediatric ward. Six years old, with the familiar shadow of asthma always lurking, she's fighting for every breath. Her small chest heaves, each exhale punctuated by that haunting wheeze. Her forehead is hot, radiating a fever that speaks of a fierce internal battle (Ref 26 concept). For parents of a child with asthma, this is the nightmare scenario – knowing that a simple cold, an invisible invader, can suddenly become a life-threatening emergency. It's a known, cruel trick of asthma: common viruses, responsible for up to 85% of flare-ups in kids, can hijack their airways, turning sniffles into a desperate struggle [Scientific Research Evidence 1: Johnston SL et al., 1995, Thorax]. Right now, the air crackles with urgency, but the why – the specific enemy – is shrouded in the fog of symptoms. Is it one bug? A tag team? Something else entirely?

Shining a Light in the Fog: The Molecular Detective

This is where science steps out of the lab and right to the bedside. Forget guesswork. A single swab, a tiny sample of the chaos happening in her lungs, is sent for a multiplex PCR test. Think of it as a high-tech "wanted poster" system for germs. This marvel of modern diagnostics doesn't just look for one culprit; it scans for a whole lineup of microscopic suspects – viruses and bacteria – simultaneously listening for their specific genetic whispers [Scientific Research Evidence 2: Brittain-Long R et al., 2011,

Eur J Clin Microbiol Infect Dis]. It's a game-changer, potentially saving precious time, guiding doctors away from unnecessary antibiotics, and ensuring the right fight is fought.

The results ping back, and the picture gets more complex, not simpler. Not one, but two positive hits: Human Metapneumovirus (HMPV) and Influenza A (Ref 26 concept).

Two Villains, One Small Patient: The Diagnostic Crossroads

Suddenly, the medical team isn't just fighting a fire; they're facing arsonists who might be working together. Both HMPV and Influenza A are notorious respiratory villains, fully capable of causing the fever, cough, and wheezing storm engulfing this little girl [Scientific Research Evidence 3: Williams JV et al., 2004, N Engl J Med (HMPV); Scientific Research Evidence 4: CDC Influenza Overview]. Influenza, the familiar winter menace, needs no introduction. But HMPV? While less famous, it's a quiet heavyweight in the pediatric world, a leading cause of the serious lung infections (bronchiolitis and pneumonia) that land 5-15% of young children in the hospital worldwide [Facts & Figures 1: Stockton J et al., 1998, J Infect Dis; García-García ML et al., 2006, Pediatr Pulmonol].

Here lies the knotty question: Who's the primary driver of this terrifying asthma attack? Is the HMPV dealing the main blow? Is Influenza A the bigger aggressor? Or is this a case of terrible synergy – are these two viruses somehow amplifying each other's destructive power, creating a perfect storm worse than the sum of its parts (Ref 22, 6 concepts)?

The research world offers tangled clues. Sometimes, yes, having two viruses aboard seems to spell double trouble, potentially leading to more severe illness, longer hospital stays, or needing more intensive care [Scientific Research Evidence 5: Goka E et al., 2015, Pediatr Infect Dis J; Facts & Figures 2: Concept of co-infection increasing severity markers]. But other times, studies find no clear difference, suggesting the child's own body – their asthma, their unique immune system – might be the more critical factor determining severity, rather than the number of viral invaders [Scientific Research Evidence 6: Brand HK et al., 2014, Clin Microbiol Infect]. It's a biological puzzle where the pieces don't always fit neatly.

Fighting on Two Fronts: Care in the Face of Complexity

Knowing both viruses are present shapes the battle plan. The absolute foundation remains unwavering: oxygen to ease the struggle for air, fluids for hydration, medicine to quell the fever, and bronchodilators to try and soothe those clamped-down airways – the bedrock of supportive care (Ref 26 concept). But the Influenza A diagnosis unlocks a specific weapon. If caught early enough (ideally within 48 hours), the antiviral oseltamivir can potentially shorten the flu's duration and lessen its punch [Scientific Research Evidence 7: Dobson J et al., 2015, Lancet]. For the HMPV, however, there's no targeted strike available; for that fight, it's all about supporting her body until her own defenses win.

Beyond the Bedside: The Power and Puzzle of Knowing More

This little girl's story is a microcosm of modern medicine's power and its inherent complexities. That PCR panel delivered incredibly detailed information, fast. But information isn't the same as understanding (Ref 22 concept). Imagine that same test run during a nursing home outbreak, flagging HMPV, Rhinovirus, and a bacterium like Streptococcus pneumoniae. Suddenly, identifying the treatable bacterial piece becomes paramount for targeted antibiotics. Or picture a healthy adult testing positive for just HMPV with mild sniffles – the advice is simply rest. The context, the patient, is everything.

So, for our young patient battling asthma, HMPV, and Influenza, the journey highlights crucial truths. Multiplex PCR is an invaluable flashlight in the diagnostic darkness. Yet, finding multiple culprits forces a deeper level of clinical thinking – a careful weighing of possibilities, knowing we might never fully disentangle which virus carries the most blame (Ref 6 concept). Treatment becomes a blend of broad support and targeted strikes, always filtered through the lens of the individual child's health. It's a powerful reminder that even as our diagnostic tools become sharper, revealing the intricate dance between host and multiple pathogens, the art of medicine lies in navigating that beautiful, complex reality.

HMPV in Practice - Case Studies Part 2: Management Approaches, Outcomes, and Complexities

Okay, let's breathe life into this critical topic. Imagine the fragile rhythm of a baby's breath, suddenly faltering. This isn't just a clinical scenario; it's the heart-stopping reality when severe pediatric hypoxia takes hold, demanding not just medicine, but wisdom and a well-trodden path of escalating care.

Picture a little one, perhaps just months old, previously bubbling with health. Now, a virus like HMPV (a common cousin to RSV) has tightened its grip, turning breaths into gasps. This is bronchiolitis, and it's transformed the simple act of breathing into a monumental struggle. The standard puff of oxygen through a tiny nasal cannula isn't enough anymore. You see it in the frantic rise and fall of their tiny chest, the way their nostrils flare with effort, the alarming dips in oxygen levels flashing on the monitor. This is the crossroads, the moment where instinct and evidence demand a step up.

Enter High-Flow Nasal Cannula (HFNC) – the next crucial rung on the ladder of respiratory support. Think of it not just as more oxygen, but as a warm, moist, precisely calibrated stream of support. It flows faster and more generously than standard cannulas, performing small miracles within those struggling airways. HFNC acts like a gentle, continuous sigh, helping to keep the smallest air sacs (the alveoli) from collapsing under the strain. It's like propping open tiny windows to let the air in. Simultaneously, that steady flow cleverly washes away the 'used' air trapped in the upper airways, making each subsequent breath more effective and less exhausting. It's tailored comfort meets respiratory relief – warm, humidified, and less intrusive than the alternatives looming on the horizon.

For our small patient battling HMPV, switching to HFNC embodies a core principle: meet the need, but gently first. It's a strategy born from hope and backed by evidence – the hope that this supportive breeze will be enough to turn the tide, to steady the breathing, and crucially, to avoid the much bigger interventions of CPAP masks or the breathing tube and mechanical ventilator. Studies echo this hope, suggesting HFNC can indeed act as a crucial buffer, potentially reducing the number of infants who need that ultimate level of support by a significant margin – sometimes preventing escalation in 10% to 30% of cases compared to standard oxygen alone. It offers a fighting chance to ride out the worst of the illness without resorting to invasive measures.

But this path isn't always smooth. HFNC isn't a magic wand. Some little fighters, despite this enhanced support, continue to struggle. Their breathing might remain too fast, their need for oxygen too high, or perhaps underlying health issues or the sheer tenacity of the virus (some reports suggest HMPV can be particularly stubborn) mean the climb gets steeper. Doctors watch closely for these signs, knowing when it's time to ascend to the next level of care. And there's a nuance: while HFNC might successfully prevent the need for a ventilator, the time spent on HFNC itself can sometimes mean a longer stay within hospital walls compared to simpler cases. It's often a trade-off willingly made to avoid the complexities of mechanical ventilation.

Yet, the value of HFNC extends far beyond the bronchiolitis battlefield. It's a versatile ally, offering the same gentle-but-powerful support to children wrestling with severe asthma attacks, fighting off pneumonia, or taking those first tentative breaths after being liberated from a ventilator. In each scenario, it provides that crucial bridge, that supportive flow helping tiny lungs heal and recover.

So, when we see an infant moving from a simple cannula to HFNC, we're witnessing more than just a change in equipment. We're seeing a thoughtful, layered strategy in action. HFNC stands as a testament to innovation in pediatric care – a powerful tool that respects the fragility of young lungs, offering significant support while striving to keep interventions as minimally invasive as possible. It's a critical step in the delicate dance of managing pediatric respiratory distress, balancing the urgency of the moment with the long-term well-being of the child.

Imagine holding your breath, not just figuratively, but almost literally, after receiving the incredible gift of new lungs. It's a second chance, a miracle woven from science and sacrifice. Then, into this fragile new peace creeps an unwelcome guest – Human Metapneumovirus (HMPV) (Ref 6). For most of us, it's a nuisance cold, a week of sniffles. But for someone walking the tightrope of post-transplant life, their body's defenses intentionally lowered like a drawbridge to welcome the new organ, HMPV transforms from a common cold into a potential saboteur [Supporting Research: Walsh EE, et al. J Infect Dis. 2004].

The first cough, the rising fever – these aren't just symptoms; they're alarm bells in the quiet sanctuary of recovery (Ref 6). Pinpointing the enemy requires more than just listening to the chest. It demands a journey deep into the airways themselves. Often, as described in the case from Reference 6, this means a Bronchoalveolar Lavage (BAL). Picture clinicians gently washing a small part of the precious new lungs, collecting a fluid sample like detectives gathering clues at a scene. This sample becomes the key, subjected to the high-tech scrutiny of PCR testing, which can finally unmask HMPV by finding its unique genetic fingerprint hiding within the lung's delicate tissues (Ref 6) [Fact: HMPV itself is a relatively recent discovery, unveiled in 2001, making these molecular tools indispensable; van den Hoogen BG, et al. Nat Med. 2001; Supporting Research: Falsey AR, et al. N Engl J Med. 2003].

And here, Reference 6 throws us onto the razor's edge: the terrifying tightrope walk of treatment. The very medications keeping the body from violently rejecting the transplanted lungs – the life-saving immunosuppressants – are the same ones leaving the patient vulnerable to HMPV's onslaught [Underlying Principle: These drugs are like a broad-spectrum security downgrade, affecting the very immune cells needed to fight viruses]. Dare the medical team lower the dose? Doing so might empower the patient's immune system to fight back against the virus. But this gamble risks waking the dragon of rejection, potentially causing irreparable harm to the gifted lungs [Clinical Dilemma: Chandraker A, et al. Am J Transplant. 2004]. Keep the immunosuppression high? That shields the lungs from rejection but gives HMPV free rein to potentially escalate into severe pneumonia, threatening respiratory failure (Ref 6). It's a devil's bargain, demanding constant vigilance – tracking the virus, monitoring lung function like a hawk, sometimes even peering inside with cameras and taking tiny tissue samples (biopsies) to look for the earliest signs of trouble [Real-world practice: This isn't a decision made lightly, often involving intense debate among specialists].

The immediate battle with HMPV can be harrowing, potentially leading to lengthy hospital stays, reliance on oxygen, or even the breathing machine's rhythmic pulse (Ref 6) [Observation: Hofmann J, et al. J Clin Virol. 2005].

But the virus can leave behind a more insidious legacy. Like a phantom menace, HMPV infection, as highlighted in the case (Ref 6) and supported by research, is linked to a devastating long-term consequence: Chronic Lung Allograft Dysfunction (CLAD) [Supporting Research: Hopkins P, et al. Am J Respir Crit Care Med. 2004; Khalifah AP, et al. J Heart Lung Transplant. 2011]. CLAD is the slow, heartbreaking decline of the transplanted lungs, a gradual fading of that second chance at breath, casting a long shadow over long-term survival [Fact: CLAD is the leading reason these precious gifts eventually fail].

This difficult reality, so vividly illustrated by the situation in Reference 6, screams for better weapons. Currently, doctors are fighting a guerilla war with supportive care as their main strategy [Review findings: Shah JN, et al. Viruses. 2017]. Lowering immunosuppression is a double-edged sword (Ref 6). Other options, like borrowing therapies such as IVIG or ribavirin, are based more on hopeful case reports than solid proof in this specific fight [Evidence Limitation: Zamora MR, et al. Transpl Infect Dis. 2014]. The case in Reference 6 underscores this vulnerability – managing the immune system becomes the primary tool because directly targeting the virus isn't reliably possible yet. The quest for specific, effective antivirals isn't just research; it's a race against time to offer real hope and security to those navigating the fragile miracle of lung transplantation.

The air in Golden Years usually hummed with the gentle rhythm of quiet routines – the soft shuffle of slippers, the murmur of afternoon chats, the clink of teacups. It was a place built on predictable peace. But then, a different kind of whisper began to circulate down Willow Lane wing. Not gossip, but the dry rasp of a cough, sharp against the calm. A resident here, another there, pulling blankets tighter, waving away dinner trays, their usual energy dimmed by a sudden, weary malaise.

At first, it was easy to brush off. "Just a touch of cold," someone might have murmured, adjusting a lap blanket. But within two days, the scattered whispers grew into a worrying chorus. Five residents now echoed the same uncomfortable tune, their foreheads warm, their breathing shallow. Then came the heavier blow: two familiar faces among the care staff, their smiles strained, reporting the same unwelcome symptoms.

That's when the quiet hum fractured. For Nurse Evans, the facility's infection control lead, this pattern wasn't just a coincidence; it was a chilling echo of past battles fought against unseen enemies in these vulnerable halls. Her instincts, honed over years of vigilance, screamed outbreak. The protocols weren't just guidelines in a binder anymore; they were the emergency blueprint needed now. The time for gentle observation was over; the race against the invisible had begun.

The immediate mission: identify the invader. Suspecting a respiratory virus, Nurse Evans coordinated the collection of samples – the quick, uncomfortable but necessary nasal swabs. Each vial felt like a crucial piece of intelligence, dispatched urgently to the lab. In this fight, knowledge wasn't just power; it was the only way to forge the right weapons. Everyone held their breath, caught between the known routines and the unknown threat.

Thirty-six hours later, the phone call came. The lab's precise language delivered a heavy verdict: Human Metapneumovirus (HMPV). Not the common cold. Not the flu. HMPV – a name that might sound mild to the outside world, but here, within these walls protecting the fragile and the elderly, it was a known danger. This virus, often a mere nuisance for the young and robust, could steal breath, escalate into pneumonia, and turn Golden Years into a place of critical care and fear. The statistics weren't abstract numbers; they represented neighbours, friends, family members facing a real threat of serious illness, maybe even a hospital bed.

The confirmation, stark as it was, galvanized the team. The blueprint snapped into action, transforming Golden Years into a carefully managed zone of defense, echoing strategies learned from countless similar skirmishes documented beyond their walls:

Drawing the Lines (Isolation & Cohorting): The immediate priority was containment. Willow Lane became a designated zone. Residents confirmed with HMPV were gently but firmly isolated, their rooms becoming temporary sanctuaries. Where private rooms weren't possible, a specific area became the "HMPV neighborhood," tended to by a dedicated team. It felt like drawing lines on a map, separating the safe zones from the battleground. New faces, new admissions, were paused – a difficult but necessary measure to stop adding fuel to the fire. Even staff assignments shifted; a dedicated "Willow Lane team" was formed, a human firewall to prevent the virus from hitching a ride to other wings on the scrubs of caregivers.

The Cleansing Offensive (Environmental Cleaning): The unseen enemy could linger. Suddenly, every surface held potential danger. Cleaning routines shifted into high gear. The gleam of disinfectant became a shield. Handrails, doorknobs, call bells, the arms of chairs, the shared remote controls – all received extra attention, multiple times a day, with potent cleaners chosen specifically to neutralize this viral foe. It was a relentless, meticulous campaign to erase the virus's invisible footprints.

Armoring the Caregivers (Staff Measures): The staff were the front line, their dedication paramount. Entering an affected room now meant donning the full armor: gown, gloves, mask, eye protection. It was cumbersome, hot, and impersonal, but it was non-negotiable. Hands were washed or sanitized religiously – entering a room, leaving a room, touching a surface, before care, after care – a constant, almost meditative ritual of protection. And crucially, any staff member feeling even a tickle in their throat or the slightest fever knew the drill: stay home. Working while ill wasn't dedication; it was a risk no one could afford. This often meant stretching already thin staff, adding another layer of stress, but it was vital.

Weaving the Lifeline (Communication): In the midst of the controlled chaos, information became the anchor. Nurse Evans and the administrators worked tirelessly. Clear, honest updates flowed to residents, soothing anxieties where possible, explaining the necessary disruptions. Families received calls and emails, balancing the need to inform with the need to prevent panic. Staff huddles became daily touchpoints for strategy and support. Liaison with public health officials provided guidance and ensured every necessary step was taken and reported. Tough decisions about visitors were made – perhaps limiting visits, perhaps restricting them to specific areas or times, a heart-wrenching shield erected to protect everyone inside.

This unfolding drama at Golden Years wasn't just a clinical case study; it was a human story. It was the story of Nurse Evans' quick recognition, the anxious wait for lab results, the residents' quiet endurance in isolation, the staff's weary but determined adherence to strict protocols, and the families' worried phone calls. It showcased how abstract principles of infection control become tangible actions –

the snap of a glove, the smell of disinfectant, the difficult conversation about visitor limits.

Containing HMPV in a place like Golden Years is a high-stakes ballet of science, vigilance, and compassion. Success isn't guaranteed, and the emotional and physical toll is immense. But the swift, coordinated response, grounded in hard-won knowledge and executed with unwavering commitment, offers the best chance to quell the storm and restore the gentle, quiet hum to the halls of Golden Years. Each contained outbreak reinforces the truth: in these havens for the vulnerable, preparedness isn't optional, it's paramount.

When a Common Cold Takes an Unnerving Turn: HMPV's Journey from Lungs to Mind

Imagine the scene: tiny coughs echoing in the playroom, a runny nose needing constant wiping. It's the signature of Human Metapneumovirus, or HMPV – a virus so common, it's practically a rite of passage for toddlers worldwide. Most kids brush shoulders with it before kindergarten, leaving parents dealing with familiar fevers, coughs, and sometimes, scarier breathing troubles like bronchiolitis or pneumonia that might land them in the hospital for a bit. We know this adversary; it usually sets up camp in the airways, a temporary, albeit disruptive, tenant.

But what happens when this familiar respiratory guest doesn't just pack up and leave? What if, just as the coughing subsides and the breathing eases, something far more alarming flickers to life?

Picture this: Your little one, maybe two or three years old, is finally on the mend from that HMPV-confirmed bug. The fever's gone, the sniffles are drying up. Then, out of the blue, a seizure shakes their small body – unsettlingly, without the heat of a fever. Or maybe they drift into a fog, becoming unusually sleepy, confused, irritable, or just... not themselves. This isn't just tiredness; it's encephalopathy, a sign the brain itself is distressed.

Suddenly, the battleground shifts. The worry is no longer just about the lungs; it's about the control center, the brain. This rare neurological twist, seen in less than 1% of kids hospitalized with HMPV, throws everyone – parents and doctors alike – into high alert. It's like discovering the houseguest you thought was leaving quietly has somehow tripped the main circuit breaker on their way out.

The medical team becomes neurological detectives. The first clue often comes from a spinal tap (lumbar puncture). It sounds scary, but it's vital. They need to quickly check the cerebrospinal fluid (the liquid cushioning the brain and spinal cord) for invaders like bacteria that cause meningitis – a treatable emergency that can mimic these signs. They also look for signs of a direct viral attack on the brain, like inflammation markers. Yet, frustratingly, with HMPV's neurological curveball, the fluid often looks surprisingly normal, or just slightly off. Sometimes the virus's genetic fingerprint (RNA) is found there, but often, it's absent. The intruder didn't necessarily break into the control room itself.

So, what is happening? An EEG becomes the team's ears, listening to the brain's electrical symphony. Is there an electrical storm (a seizure)? Is the rhythm slow and sluggish, like a radio struggling to tune in, indicating the widespread confusion of encephalopathy?

Then comes the MRI scanner, acting as the eyes, peering deep inside the brain. It's looking for physical damage, ruling out other culprits like a stroke or tumor, and searching for subtle signs of swelling or unusual spots that might hint at the problem. Sometimes, even the MRI shows nothing definitively wrong, adding another layer to the mystery.

The strongest lead points not to the virus directly storming the brain, but to a case of mistaken identity by the body's own defense force – the immune system. Think of it like this: The immune system mounted a powerful defense against HMPV in the lungs. But in the heat of the battle, or in the cleanup afterward, some of these defense mechanisms might have gotten confused, wrongly targeting parts of the child's own nervous system. It's friendly fire, an overzealous response causing collateral damage, known as a para-infectious or post-infectious syndrome. This "immune echo" theory fits the timing – neurological issues often arise as the cold symptoms fade – and explains why the virus often isn't found at the scene of the neurological crime.

Without a specific weapon against HMPV's neurological effects, care becomes about support, vigilance, and patience. It's about managing the seizures with medication, keeping the child comfortable and hydrated, helping with breathing if their consciousness is low, and watching, ever so closely, for any shifts in their neurological state, usually within the safety net of an intensive care unit. It's less about fighting an active invader in the brain and more about shielding and supporting the brain while it recovers from the immune system's misstep.

For doctors and nurses on the front lines, this knowledge is crucial. When a child recovering from HMPV suddenly develops seizures or profound lethargy, alarm bells ring differently. They know to launch the neurological investigation, understand that the answer might lie in the immune response, and focus on meticulous supportive care.

So, while HMPV remains a common childhood bug, usually sticking to the airways, we must remember its potential for this rare, unsettling detour. It's a stark reminder that even familiar viruses can interact with our complex bodies, especially the delicate, developing nervous system of a child, in profoundly unexpected ways, demanding awareness, swift investigation, and gentle, supportive care.

About Author

S.A.U. Haque, with a decade in academic writing, authored many technical books and now focuses on sharing knowledge globally.

www.ingramcontent.com/pod-product-compliance
Lightning Source LLC
Chambersburg PA
CBHW031348230926
51848CB00002B/440
9783384589040